"One of the most difficult tasks faced
patients to engage in positive behaviors such as maintaining a ....
Gould, and Strosahl's *Real Behavior Change in Primary Care* adds ACT to
the growing list of techniques that are available to help the primary care
provider convince patients to change their behaviors for the better. In simple,
readable prose, they outline a strategy with wide implications for improving
primary care practice."

—Robert McGrath, PhD, professor of psychology at
Fairleigh Dickinson University

"The authors have provided an outstanding set of assessment and intervention tools that primary care providers can use with patients who are stuck
in maladaptive health patterns. The downloadable tools, practical advice,
and focused clinical examples can be easily incorporated into everyday practice, leading to better patient outcomes, decreased provider burnout, and
increased job satisfaction."

—Christopher L. Hunter, PhD, ABPP, coauthor of
Integrated Behavioral Health in Primary Care

"This book is a tremendous resource to primary care providers and providers
of behavioral health in primary care. Readers can expect greater satisfaction
in seeing their patients reach positive health outcomes. Our organization is
appreciative to the authors for enhancing both the career satisfaction of our
providers and the quality of care our patients receive."

—Bill Rosenfeld, LPC, director of integrated behavioral
health at Mountain Park Health Center

"*Real Behavior Change in Primary Care* is succinct, practical, and easy to read. It provides the primary care clinician with a fresh view of the complex patient and an array of tools that are easy to implement in a busy clinic, even without a psychotherapy background. The techniques offered can help primary care providers improve management of the complex patient while also healing themselves of the frustration and stress that can accompany a caseload of challenging patients. The authors' values-driven approach to care is neither paternalistic nor unrealistic. Rather, it supports providers and patients in developing activities congruent with personal values and life directions. I enjoyed reading the book and will be using the techniques illustrated with my patients, my medical and psychology trainees, and myself!"

> —Jeannie A. Sperry, PhD, associate professor and director
> of behavior science education at West Virginia University
> Department of Family Medicine

"The authors have adapted the latest advances in evidence-based behavioral and cognitive therapies for use in the fast-paced primary care environment. The straightforward explanations, rich array of resources, and practical handouts are immediately beneficial for helping patients live life in a way that is more consistent with their values. Many primary care providers may particularly appreciate the authors' discussion of how to self-apply ACT interventions to reduce burnout and become reinvigorated with patient care and other valued life activities. This book is an essential resource for any primary care provider working to help patients change what they do and how they think."

> —Jeffrey L. Goodie, PhD, ABPP, clinical health psychologist
> at Uniformed Services University of Health Sciences
> in Bethesda, MD, and coauthor of *Integrated Behavioral
> Health in Primary Care*

Real Behavior

Change in

Primary Care

IMPROVING PATIENT OUTCOMES &
INCREASING JOB SATISFACTION

PATRICIA J. ROBINSON, PhD
DEBRA A. GOULD, MD, MPH
KIRK D. STROSAHL, PhD

New Harbinger Publications, Inc.

Publisher's Note

This publication is designed to provide accurate and authoritative information in regard to the subject matter covered. It is sold with the understanding that the publisher is not engaged in rendering psychological, financial, legal, or other professional services. If expert assistance or counseling is needed, the services of a competent professional should be sought.

Distributed in Canada by Raincoast Books

Copyright © 2010 by Patricia J. Robinson, Debra A. Gould, & Kirk D. Strosahl
New Harbinger Publications, Inc.
5674 Shattuck Avenue
Oakland, CA 94609
www.newharbinger.com

Cover design by Amy Shoup
Text design by Tracy Marie Carlson
Acquired by Catharine Sutker
Edited by Nelda Street

The Library of Congress has cataloged the hardcover edition as:

Robinson, Patricia J.
  Real behavior change in primary care : improving patient outcomes and increasing job satisfaction / Patricia J. Robinson, Debra A. Gould, and Kirk D. Strosahl.
     p. ; cm.
  Includes bibliographical references and index.
  ISBN 978-1-57224-832-8 (pbk.) -- ISBN 978-1-57224-833-5 (pdf ebook) 1. Clinical health psychology. 2. Acceptance and commitment therapy. 3. Health behavior. 4. Primary care (Medicine) I. Gould, Debra A. II. Strosahl, Kirk, 1950- III. Title.
  [DNLM: 1. Cognitive Therapy--methods. 2. Burnout, Professional--prevention & control. 3. Patient Compliance--psychology. 4. Patients--psychology. 5. Physicians, Family--psychology. 6. Primary Health Care--trends. WM 425.5.C6]
  R726.7.R625 2010
  616.001'9--dc22
                              2010043965

20   19   18
10   9   8   7   6   5   4

To Dr. Kay Funk, who encouraged me to write this book; to Dr. Mark Sauerwein, who encouraged me to teach; and to all the other wise people I have known who committed their lives to providing primary care.

—Patti

To Michael Joseph Aquilino for his unconditional love and support in making all of this possible, to ZaChoeje Rinpoche for his brilliance, to Leslie Gray for starting me on this path, and to my mother Vera Rock Gould, who always told me that if I could read a book, I could learn how to do anything.

—Deb

To my brother (and Patti's brother-in-law), Mark Strosahl; we wish you were here to read this book, as with the other books. We miss you, buddy—every day, in every way.

—Kirk (and Patti)

Contents

Acknowledgments ix

Introduction 1

PART 1
A New Model for Addressing Psychological Problems

CHAPTER 1
Beyond Mind as a Machine 11

CHAPTER 2
How People Get Stuck 29

CHAPTER 3
Creating a Context for Change 39

CHAPTER 4
Takin' It to the Streets: Real Behavior Change Tools 61

PART 2
Promoting Real Behavior
Change in Patient Care

CHAPTER 5
The Struggle: Engaging Patients with Chronic Disease... 87

CHAPTER 6
The Solution That Becomes the Problem:
Intervening with Alcohol and Substance Abuse 103

CHAPTER 7
"Doc, This Pain Is Killing Me":
Addressing Chronic Pain with Compassion............ 119

CHAPTER 8
A Fresh Approach to the Daily Duo:
Anxiety and Depression..................... 137

CHAPTER 9
Living in the Past, Dying in the Present:
Trauma and Violence 155

PART 3
Applying Real Behavior Change
Tools in Daily Practice

CHAPTER 10
Better and Faster: The Risk of Burnout 177

CHAPTER 11
Provider Wellness: Preventing Burnout and
Improving Job Satisfaction...................... 193

APPENDIX A
Acceptance and Action Questionnaire (AAQ-II) 205

APPENDIX B
Primary Care Provider Acceptance and
Action Questionnaire (PCP-AAQ) 207

APPENDIX C
Primary Care Provider Stress Checklist (PCP-SC) 210

APPENDIX D
Real Behavior Change Interviewing—The Three-T
and Workability Questions 215

APPENDIX E
Real Behavior Change Interviewing—
The Love, Work, Play, and Health Questions 216

APPENDIX F
Six Core Processes—Psychological Flexibility 218

APPENDIX G
Core Process Assessment Tool (CPAT) 219

APPENDIX H
Real Behavior Change Pocket Guide 221

APPENDIX I
Patient Education—Bull's-Eye Worksheet 224

APPENDIX J
Provider Tool—Retirement Party Worksheet.......... 226

APPENDIX K
Provider Tool—Bull's-Eye Professional and
Personal Values Assessment 227

APPENDIX L
Burnout Prevention and Recovery Plan 228

References 229

Index... 241

Acknowledgments

We would like to express our appreciation for New Harbinger's willingness to make a bold move in publishing a book for primary care providers. We would also like to thank our clinical and research colleagues at Group Health Cooperative of Seattle, for supporting our initial exploration of primary care behavioral health integration. Coworkers at Yakima Valley Farm Workers Clinics (Patti) and Central Washington Family Medicine (Kirk) have contributed in numerous ways to the creation of this work. Of special mention, of course, is Deb Gould, who has worked tenaciously to help us translate the newest cognitive and behavioral interventions into a language and format for primary care. Dozens of other primary care providers in community health centers throughout the United States and in military medical treatment facilities around the world have also shaped our thinking. Physicians and nurses in the Veteran's Administration medical system, numerous health maintenance organization (HMO) systems, and providers in individual medical practices have also listened to us and evaluated and refined our thinking. Most recently, we've had the privilege of working with many capable primary care providers in San Francisco Department of Public Health clinics. We offer gratitude beyond words to all of these physicians, midlevel providers, nurses, and their primary care behavioral health colleagues. Last (and maybe they should have been first), we acknowledge the thousands of primary care patients who have been our daily teachers over the past thirty-five years. Patients, we thank you for your transparency, your patience, your trust, and your willingness to engage in behavior change and pursuit of a more meaningful life!

—Patti and Kirk

I would like to thank Patti and Kirk for their patience and willingness to teach me how to apply ACT in my daily practice and to include me in this wonderful project. I would also like to thank the faculty, staff, and colleagues at Highland Hospital/University of Rochester Family Medicine Residency for the excellent training in psychosocial and evidence-based medicine that set the stage for my ability to incorporate ACT into patient care. Thanks also to Tom Taylor, MD, Ph.D., at the University of Washington–Seattle, for his unconditional mentoring. Many thanks also go to Central Washington Family Medicine Residency Administration for incorporating the primary care behavioral health model into our care of patients and giving me the opportunity to work side by side with Kirk Strosahl. And last but not least, my heartfelt thanks go to my patients, who make this work meaningful.

—Deb

Introduction

As two psychologists and a physician, we live, eat, and breathe primary care medicine. Our roles include practicing in primary care (PC), teaching family medicine residents and PC behavioral health providers, conducting practice-based research, and consulting with health care systems. We wrote this book with the hope of providing a new perspective on practicing medicine in the primary care setting. These very troubling times for medicine affect you, regardless of whether you are a medical doctor, doctor of osteopathy, nurse practitioner, physician assistant, registered nurse, or student in a medical school or nursing program. The health care system is broken, and most health care providers are being asked to do more in less time and for less pay. Every year, record numbers of graduating medical students turn their backs on a career in general medicine, electing instead to practice a medical subspecialty or practice in a hospital setting. They have heard that primary care is a fast and furious setting, with high levels of work stress and relatively low pay compared to a subspecialization.

At the same time, a virtual pandemic of human suffering is going on, ranging from unprecedented rates of mental disorders and addictions to conditions resulting from unhealthy lifestyles (for example, obesity, lung disease, STDs), pain syndromes, and poor to nonexistent self-management of chronic disease. Health care providers address most of these problems on a day-in, day-out basis. Apart from prescribing drugs, health care providers often feel at a loss as to how to help their patients change unworkable, health-threatening behaviors. Fresh ideas are needed if we are to find better solutions to the practice-related factors that contribute to work stress, job dissatisfaction, and burnout. Clearly, one of these stresses is the pressure to help patients who are suffering, in the context of limited time and resources to do so. This book will help you manage that pressure and, at the same time, help you provide better care to your patients. The approach recommended in the book has a track record for identifying medical providers who are at risk for burnout (Losa Iglesias, Becerro de Bengoa Vallejo, & Salvadores Fuentes, 2010), inspiring interventions that can enhance resiliency in human service workers (Hayes, Bissett, et al., 2004), and helping providers obtain better outcomes with patients who can be difficult to treat in primary care (Forman, Herbert, Moitra, Yeomans, & Geller, 2007; Gregg, Callaghan, Hayes, & Glenn-Lawson, 2007; Gifford et al., 2004; Hayes, Wilson, et al., 2004; Hayes, Luoma, Bond, Masuda, & Lillis, 2006; Lundgren, Dahl, Yardi, & Melin, 2008; McCracken & Eccleston, 2003; Zettle & Rains, 1989). Read on to learn ways to provide more-effective care to patients *and* to reduce your stress as a medical care provider.

The model we describe represents a shift from overreliance on the bio-medical model of human suffering to using a contextual framework to understand and treat suffering in all of its forms. Because medical and nursing students are not normally exposed to contextual models of behavior change, some of this material may seem quite new and possibly even counterintuitive. At the same time, some of the messages that emanate from the contextual model are timeless and have worked their way into the fabric of contemporary society. As you read this book, you may notice that you have applied some of these principles in your own life.

THE PROBLEM OF CHANGING HUMAN BEHAVIOR

Several earlier works have attempted to grapple with addressing behavioral health problems in very short medical encounters. Classics such as *The Fifteen-Minute Hour* (Stuart & Lieberman, 2002) and *Field Guide to the Difficult Patient Interview* (Platt & Gordon, 1999) have been extremely valuable in describing patient-centered interview techniques and evidence-based intervention strategies for specific conditions. In the tradition of standing on the shoulders of giants, what we believe is missing is an overarching framework for assessment and intervention that can be applied regardless of what the human problem is—in essence, a unified model of human suffering and how to address it in a fifteen-minute medical exam.

In this book, our aim is to provide you with a conceptual framework for addressing the myriad types of behavioral health problems you will see, rather than give you a cookbook approach that requires you to memorize a different set of interventions for each of the two dozen problems you see every day. In the world of primary care, we need simplification that does not result in a loss of effectiveness and that simultaneously supports creativity in our interventions. The approach we use is called acceptance and commitment therapy (or ACT, pronounced like the verb "act"), and we intend to teach you to use this model to help you reduce your patients' suffering and create balance in your own life.

Like motivational interviewing (Miller & Rollnick, 2002) and mindfulness-based stress reduction (Grossman, Niemann, Schmidt, & Walach, 2004), ACT offers primary care providers new tools to improve patient outcomes and enhance provider and patient satisfaction. In the case of motivational interviewing, primary care providers learn to steer away from lecturing patients on their unhealthy habits and outcomes and to focus instead on matching appropriate psychosocial tools to the patient's level of readiness for change. Mindfulness-based stress reduction techniques help us teach patients to be aware and accepting of their experience in the moment. ACT offers a variety of new tools, plus a new conceptual framework. With ACT interventions, patients learn to become more aware of avoidant behavior patterns that cost them vitality in living. They also learn to be more "present" in their lives and to choose behavioral directions according to their values. ACT is about acceptance, choice, commitment, and taking action. The role of the primary care provider is unique, and the opportunities inherent in building relationships with patients over a lifetime are rich indeed. It is from this strategic position that providers of primary care can provide a sustained effort to help patients apply ACT techniques and move toward value-consistent action over time.

EVIDENCE FOR ACT

ACT is a relatively new form of cognitive behavioral therapy (CBT), but there is already promising research on its application in the primary care setting (Hayes, Strosahl, & Wilson, 1999). One of the most exciting studies involved using ACT with patients with diabetes. Compared with patients receiving the usual care, ACT patients had better self-reported diabetes management and significant improvement in hemoglobin A1c measurement (Gregg, Callaghan, Hayes, & Glenn-Lawson, 2007). In another study, patients receiving an ACT intervention demonstrated improved rates of smoking cessation (Gifford et al., 2004). Studies conducted in Sweden and the United Kingdom suggest that ACT is a powerful treatment for chronic pain and disability behavior (McCracken & Eccleston, 2003; Dahl, Wilson, & Nilsson, 2004). ACT strategies have been shown to reduce the rate of seizures and improve quality of life in patients with uncontrolled seizure disorder (Lundgren et al., 2008). Research suggests that ACT interventions are also helpful to depressed patients (Zettle & Rains, 1989) and polysubstance-abusing, methadone-maintained opiate addicts (Hayes, Wilson, et al., 2004). Finally, recent meta-analyses of ACT studies have concluded that ACT is better than usual care or waiting lists and as effective as other cognitive behavioral therapies or other psychotherapies in the treatment of many traditional mental health problems commonly seen in primary care (Powers, Zum Vörde Sive Vörding, & Emmelkamp, 2009), including anxiety (Hayes et al., 2006).

While most studies on ACT have used formats more typical of traditional mental health, Kevin Vowles and his colleagues used a brief ACT intervention with patients suffering from chronic low-back pain, and they reported that patients instructed on pain acceptance performed better on a measure of physical impairment compared to patients trained on a pain control strategy and patients receiving a placebo (Vowles et al., 2007). In our practice, we use ACT in ten-, fifteen-, and twenty-five-minute visits with patients. We believe that the practice of ACT in primary care will amplify the impact of the *medical home* model, where behavioral health providers work as members of the primary care team, providing consultation services to primary care providers and primary care patients. Adopting a common behavioral health treatment philosophy across the entire primary care team will allow nurses, doctors, midlevel practitioners, on-site mental health providers, and other team members to "sing from the same sheet," to use an old adage.

For integrating behavioral health services into primary care, we use the primary care behavioral health (PCBH) model as our platform for delivering ACT interventions (see Robinson & Reiter, 2007, for guidelines on how to implement this model). This model brings a mental health provider to the primary care team, a behavioral health consultant (BHC), to assist with treatment plan development and skill training for patients with medical problems (such as obesity, hypertension, and diabetes), behavioral health problems (such as relationship problems, depression, anxiety, and traumatic stress), and combined medical and behavioral health problems (which is often the case). To demonstrate how ACT works in the PCBH model, we present several case examples involving a BHC team member in this book. However, the new primary care health care system is evolving, and not all primary care providers have the benefit of working with a BHC, so rather than assume availability of these services, our basic approach focuses on interventions traditional members of the primary care team (the physician, midlevel primary care provider, and nurse) can provide. Throughout the book, when we use the term primary care provider (PCP), we are referring to all of these traditional members of the primary care team.

ACT AND OCCUPATIONAL STRESS

It is clear that the stresses of practicing general medicine grow daily, and many indicators suggest that PCPs are feeling the strain. A recent study of intensive care nurses in Spain found a positive correlation between scores on an ACT measure of emotional avoidance (the Acceptance and Action Questionnaire) and on measures of depersonalization and emotional exhaustion on the Maslach Burnout Inventory (Losa Iglesias et al., 2010). Compared to the general population, physicians suffer from depression and abuse alcohol and drugs at least at the same rates as the general population (Center et al., 2003), and they have higher rates of suicide (Schernhammer & Colditz, 2004). ACT has been applied with considerable success to the problem of stress and burnout, not yet with physicians and nurses, but with mental health and chemical dependency therapists (Hayes, Bissett, et al., 2004). When these human service professionals learned to apply ACT in their work settings, they reported increased job satisfaction and decreased burnout.

What are the factors that contribute to provider stress and burnout? An analysis in the U.S. Physician Worklife Study suggests that solo practice, long work hours, time pressures, complex patients, less control over the workplace, interruptions, lack of support from colleagues for work–home balance, and isolation (for example, gender minority status) contribute to this large and growing problem (Linzer et al., 2002). A recent qualitative study of Canadian family physicians (Lee, Stewart, & Brown, 2008) suggested additional factors, including paperwork, new medical information, difficult patients, rules and regulations requiring more documentation, limited resources, difficulties accessing specialists (as well as diagnostic tests and community programs), and being undervalued.

Are there factors or qualities that counterbalance the negative impact of these all-too-common stresses in medical practice? Qualitative studies suggest that specific factors can provide a counterbalance and enhance resilience among family physicians (Lee, Brown, & Stewart, 2009), including being able to identify personal and psychological strategies for addressing stress, such as self-awareness and acceptance of limitations. Additionally, the ability to prioritize values is a protective factor. ACT offers a framework for PCPs to use in developing these qualities. This book attempts to offer PCPs, including residents and medical students, ACT-based methods for developing the hardiness needed to stay the course in practice.

THIS BOOK IN A NUTSHELL

This book is divided into three parts. In part 1, chapter 1 is designed to help you expand your view of human suffering, chapter 2 introduces six core ACT processes that promote suffering (Six Core Processes: Psychological Rigidity), and chapter 3 introduces six core processes that promote vitality and psychologically flexible problem solving (Six Core Processes: Psychological Flexibility). Chapter 4 concludes this part of the book by offering specific tools for interviewing for behavior change and assessing patient strengths and weaknesses in core ACT processes, a guide for selecting a specific technique to help patients develop skills indicated by assessment findings, and the Bull's-Eye Worksheet, a flexible tool for supporting patients in meaningful behavior change over time.

Offering examples of how to apply the interventions introduced in part 1, part 2 includes five chapters, each with a focus on patients who often represent challenges for PCPs. Case examples in chapters 5 through 9 include a variety of patients, and these chapters invite you to imagine the benefit of having a behavioral health provider as a team member.

In part 3, chapter 10 offers tools for assessing your risk for burnout, given your pursuit of a career replete with both positive and negative stressors.

Techniques from the Real Behavior Change Pocket Guide (also in appendix H and online) may be useful to both you and your patients. In the final chapter of the book, chapter 11, we offer several formats for building and rebuilding your resilience to stress and your connection with the values that led you to choose to work in medicine.

Clean copies of the forms most commonly used in case examples in this book are available both in the appendixes and online at http://www.newhar bingeronline.com/real-behavior-change-in-primary-care.html, including:

- Assessment forms (Acceptance and Action Questionnaire II [AAQ-II] (Bond et al., 2010), Primary Care Provider Acceptance and Action Questionnaire [PCP-AAQ], and Primary Care Provider Stress Checklist [PCP-SC])

- A case conceptualization tool (Core Process Assessment Tool [CPAT])

- A treatment planning tool (Real Behavior Change Pocket Guide)

- A behavior change tool (Bull's-Eye Worksheet, illustrated repeatedly throughout the book)

Additional forms supporting patient education and two bonus chapters ("Angry Patients and Soft Eyes: Connecting with the Help-Rejecting Patient" and "You're Okay but Not for Long: Addressing Health-Risk Behavior") are also available online.

Throughout this book, when this symbol appears next to discussions about a diagram or worksheet, you can find a copy online at http://www. newharbingeronline.com/real-behavior-change-in-primary-care.html.

HOW TO USE THIS BOOK

Your responses to the Primary Care Provider Stress Checklist (PCP-SC; appendix C and online) may help you plan your approach to reading this book. Go to the website and print the PCP-SC now, respond to the items, and use the scoring directions to help you identify your highest sources of stress. The following table will help you identify the chapters with the most pertinent information for alleviating stress. Chapters 1 through 4 provide a foundation for all readers, so read them *before* branching out to other chapters.

PCP-SC Source of Stress	Stress Score	Chapter(s) to Read
Interactions with Patients		5–9
Practice Management		10–11
Administrative Issues		10–11
Education/Learning		10–11
Relationships with Colleagues		11
Balance Between Work and the "Rest of Life"		11
Total PCP-SC Score		

CONCLUSION

We hope our introduction has sparked some curiosity in you. Indeed, whenever you believe there might be something more to understand or a new approach to an old problem, you have an opportunity to change and better your course. This book will provide you with a framework not only for viewing your patients and yourself with more levity, compassion, and acceptance, but also for resolving problems more creatively, turning a flicker of hope into a steady glow of purposeful living.

PART 1

A New Model for Addressing Psychological Problems

In this part, we provide information to help you build a strong foundation for applying real behavior change techniques in primary care. You will learn about a new view of human suffering and six core processes involved in the development of psychological rigidity and unnecessary suffering. You will also learn about six core processes that promote psychological flexibility in responding to life problems. Then, we offer you specific tools for interviewing patients, conceptualizing their strengths and weaknesses, and, finally, engaging patients in planning and pursuing more meaningful lives—the bull's-eye!

A New Model for Addressing Psychological Problems

3

CHAPTER 1

Beyond Mind as a Machine

This chapter offers you an opportunity to look at new ways to understand and deal with the human suffering you see in your medical practice. We hope to offer you a perspective on behavior change that differs significantly from your current perspective, starting with a brief history of behavioral approaches over the past hundred years and then comparing the traditional biomedical approach with a new, contextual view of suffering and change.

A BRIEF HISTORY OF BEHAVIORAL APPROACHES TO SUFFERING

Let's begin with a review of efforts to address psychological suffering in the Western world over the past century. In the early twentieth century, proponents of psychoanalysis proposed that suffering was the result of unresolved unconscious conflicts and yearnings that were not socially acceptable. Consequently, they developed procedures, such as free association and dream interpretation, to unleash the contents of the unconscious using a lexicon that included terms such as "id," "ego," "superego," "transference," and "countertransference" to describe dynamic interactions between conscious and unconscious processes. While these concepts related loosely to scientific findings, they required a great deal of time to learn and apply. Therefore, they did not become available to most patients, particularly those presenting to medical settings.

As scientific efforts to address psychological problems proceeded, behavioral approaches came to fruition. The behaviorists strove to predict and control behavior (Watson, 1913). Essentially, three rivers of work emerged from the initial stream of behaviorism. The first behaviorists focused on observation and modification of human behavior or observable actions (Wolpe, 1958). They offered principles derived from scientific, laboratory-based studies, including operant and classical conditioning, extinction, counterconditioning, and schedules of reinforcement. Behaviorists noted the importance of mental activity in psychological problems but avoided attempts to predict or control language and cognition, because direct observation of these aspects was not possible.

When computers began to play an important role in our society, scientists began to see the mind as analogous to a powerful computer, capable of processing huge amounts of information and making decisions. This model worked well in accounting for human mental abilities for solving problems in the material world, and it appeared to hold promise for understanding how human mental abilities could also address problematic thinking and emotions. Cognitive behavioral theorists led the way in this second stream of behaviorism, asserting that the cause of mental suffering was distorted, irrational thinking and poor problem-solving skills, resulting in self-defeating behaviors (see for example, Beck, 1995; D'Zurilla & Nezu, 1999; Ellis, 2001). The goal of cognitive behavioral therapy (CBT) was to teach patients to eliminate errors in thinking and develop problem-solving skills, which would presumably result in reducing or eliminating self-defeating behaviors.

CBT treatments were the first psychological treatments to be evaluated in large, well-controlled clinical trials. Typically, research described interventions in detailed treatment manuals, which then guided replication studies by other researchers. Therapists delivering experimental treatments received intense training to ensure treatment fidelity, and usual-care or wait-list control groups were employed to evaluate differential effectiveness. CBT treatments were developed and tested for many problems (such as depression, panic, OCD, and social phobia). The main outcome variable in most CBT clinical trials was reduction in symptoms of the mental disorder in question. While findings suggested that CBT treatments reduced symptoms associated with the mental disorder targeted by intervention protocol, there was little or no evidence that these protocols decreased distorted, negative thoughts. Unfortunately, these studies did not systematically measure the patient's functioning or quality of life, so we don't know how CBT affects the patient's functioning in daily life. There has been no appreciable improvement in the impact of CBT treatments since the mid-1990s, suggesting that traditional CBT has reached a plateau in terms of what it has to offer. The lack of continued improvement in outcomes produced by CBT, combined with the fact that every CBT treatment relies on the mastery of complicated treatment manuals, spawned a search for a simpler, transdiagnostic approach that might be as effective as CBT treatments.

There is some irony in the fact that the third and most recent stream of behaviorism to emerge actually goes back to the work of B. F. Skinner (1950) and to a tradition known as *behavior analysis*. In one of his last works (Skinner, 1989), Skinner speculated that human language and thought follow the same rules of learning and reinforcement as observable behavior and that the human "mind" interacts with the environment in much the same way observable behavior does. While traditional behavioral analysts rejected this idea, a small group of researchers known as "radical behaviorists" began to pursue this idea in the laboratory. Over the last fifteen years, scientists in countries all over the world have investigated a resulting behavioral analytic model of language called *relational frame theory* (RFT) and its application to a wide range of psychological problems.

RFT has illuminated the processes by which we develop thought, associate emotional arousal with thought and memories, and develop rules to direct our behavior in response to imagined events (such as *making a mistake*) and associated consequences (such as *being laughed at* or *being punished*). We can derive rules that teach us to avoid painful events, situations, or interactions (*Don't make a mistake or you'll be laughed at*) and rules that will allow us to endure immense suffering in pursuit of a valued consequence (*I will make it through medical [or nursing] school because I have a mission to help people improve their health, and that dignifies my forgoing more immediately pleasurable activities*).

There are a number of important and far-reaching clinical implications of RFT research:

- First, language and thought control human behavior, and socially inculcated rules buried within language are the "operating system." By this, we mean that language processes that often operate outside of awareness govern human behavior. Your patients are socially trained to attack life problems in particular ways, and they will respond to life problems similarly (for example, *Don't think about your diabetes and you won't feel upset; if you are not upset, then you are doing well*).

■ Second, as we shall see later in this chapter, socially inculcated rules tend to be indiscriminately applied regardless of the type of problem, and some problems may actually get worse when these strategies are used. Since these rules are nested within language, it's easy to just assume they are true and never question them.

■ Third, not surprisingly, behavior that is rule-governed in this way is not responsive to direct consequences; individuals will follow unworkable rules despite harsh results and often will *increase* the intensity of rule following in the face of negative results (for example, a patient who has suffered years of domestic violence may insist, "If I'm very careful, I won't make my husband angry and he won't be violent toward me").

■ Fourth, through the vehicle of symbolic language, patients can and do rapidly equate you with other providers and other health care situations they have been involved in previously, despite the fact that they hardly know you (for example, the chronic pain patient who just "knows" you secretly want to stop the narcotics no matter what you say) (Blackledge, 2003; Hayes, Barnes-Holmes, & Roche, 2001).

To learn more about RFT, we recommend *Learning RFT* (Törneke, 2010).

In concluding this introduction to behavioral therapies, we want to clarify that the third river of behaviorism focuses on *processes* that create human suffering, rather than on the specific symptoms of mental disorders. People express their suffering in an endless variety of ways. To use a medical analogy, these are phenotypic expressions of suffering. In the new behaviorism, we are more interested in the genotypic processes that produce all forms of suffering, because this will allow us to have a far-reaching impact on our patients. The good news is that this shift makes behavioral strategies far more flexible and easy to learn. You don't need an hour (or even fifteen minutes) to talk with a patient in ways that can promote rapid and long-lasting change (and that's what we mean by real behavior change). Now, you can efficiently apply these ACT principles in medical exams and improve patient outcomes, reduce your stress level, and improve your job satisfaction.

HUMAN SUFFERING: TWO COMPETING PERSPECTIVES

We now turn our attention to the cornerstone issue that every medical professional addresses in either a conscious or an unconscious fashion. When you see a patient who is suffering in some way, how do you account for it? Do you think suffering is an abnormal state of existence that must somehow be alleviated at any cost? Or do you see suffering as an inevitable part of human existence? The stance you take will inform what you ask the patient and what you will do to help. Next we will review two roughly opposite perspectives.

The Biomedical Approach

In the biomedical approach, a great deal of attention is paid to the "form" of the patient's complaints and symptoms. Based on the number and severity of symptoms, a "diagnosis" is made, often of some type of underlying disease process or syndrome. Symptoms are assumed to signal the existence of an underlying functional disease process, thus accurately identifying and measuring symptom severity is critical. For example, a temperature of 104 degrees surely indicates that something is amiss in the patient's body. By searching for additional symptoms, the primary care provider can make a differential diagnosis of what that process is and what treatment is indicated. This approach assumes that illness is a disruption of the body's natural homeostasis, and the goal of treatment is to manage or cure that disruptive process. Thus, to make a diagnosis of depression, the provider tabulates the number of symptoms, as well as their severity and impact, and then selects from a variety of possible mood disorder diagnoses.

At heart, the biomedical model is rooted in two different philosophies: reductionism and mechanism. *Reductionism* suggests that things are better "known" if we can break them down into small cause-and-effect relationships. For example, to understand what causes cancer, we need to discover the processes that lead to tumor formation. *Mechanism* holds that cause-and-effect relationships are rooted in the physical world and are more or less automatic. In studying the causes of cancer, the assumption is that pathogenesis occurs through a series of cause-and-effect actions that invariably disrupt the body's ability to kill off invading cells.

The mechanistic model is often applied successfully to address common physical problems (for example, antibiotics are used to eliminate pneumonia-causing bacteria). It is also useful in solving many problems in our external environment (for example, getting an air conditioner to eliminate the problem of sleeping in a very hot room). Applied to psychological suffering, mechanism suggests that something in the mind is "broken" and needs to be fixed. One popular mechanistic theory of depression is that it is the effect of irregularities in serotonin uptake at the synaptic cleft. Prescribing a medication "repairs" the parts of the brain that are presumed to be malfunctioning, consistent with the notion that depression is an illness or disease. These strategies all emanate from an assumption that we can better "know" depression if we examine its neurochemical parts, identify what is broken, and use a medical intervention to correct the abnormality.

The Contextual Approach

The *contextual* approach, often called "functional contextualism," is concerned with the *function*, rather than the form, of complaints or symptoms. A contextual assessment of depression would focus on how a patient's depressed behaviors interact with the patient's environment. For example, rather than focusing on fatigue as a "symptom" of depression, we would focus on how fatigue functions in the patient's life. Does the patient name fatigue as a "reason" for avoiding activities that might improve her energy and mood, such as exercising, going to social gatherings, or attending church? How does avoiding these activities work for the patient? Does mood or energy improve, or is the result a stronger sense of isolation and even greater problems with energy and mood? The tendency to use sensations and emotions as justifications for behavior is common in human beings, and it is problematic when it takes us away from, rather than toward, what we care about.

In a contextual approach, we focus on the interaction the patient has with his internal (mental) and external (environmental) contexts. In regard to depression, the PCP would assist the patient with developing a new perspective on "fatigue as a reason" for deciding daily activities. The PCP might ask the patient to consider short- and long-term consequences of using fatigue as the "ruler." Additionally, the PCP might ask questions to help the patient recognize the possibility of an active approach orientation to planning activities (for example, "When you were most proud of how your life was going, what did your daily routine look like?"). In a contextual approach, the emphasis is on helping the patient develop a new relationship with the problematic mental experience (such as rules that promise one thing but deliver another) and the ability to engage in approach-oriented (rather than avoidance-focused) behaviors.

As you can see from this brief discussion about treatment of depression, the contextual approach assumes that human suffering emanates from ordinary processes that are not abnormal but instead are simply not working to support the best interests of the patient. In the next section, we will delve into the everyday causes of suffering and how they manifest in the language of the patient. For now, understand that a core tenet of contextual theory is that patients are not "broken" but rather are trapped in rigid patterns of behavior that block them from pursuing more meaningful lives. For reasons we will explicate later, the patient is not "reading" these negative consequences and learning to respond in more effective ways, which is a problem health care providers see every day—for example, the patient who has had a heart attack but continues to smoke, or the patient with a drinking problem who presents for the third time with severe stomach pain. These are examples of suffering that require us to go beyond the mechanistic approach. We believe (and hope to convince you) that the contextual model is a new and powerful way to work with primary care patients who have more-complex presentations, such as patients with diabetes who have self-management skill deficits and patients with chronic pain who are demoralized by their multiple health problems.

PAIN AND SUFFERING

In ACT and other contextual behavior change approaches, we differentiate between pain and suffering. Pain is always a part of life: we are growing older, our bodies deteriorate with time, and as time passes we experience multiple positive and negative stresses. Pain, heartache, and setbacks are part of our birthright and, given the proper perspective, can be a rich source of learning and personal growth.

While pain is part of the human condition, suffering is optional. Suffering is a uniquely human attribute that originates in our ability to evaluate, categorize, compare, and predict. As children we learn to judge "good" and "bad" and to avoid being bad. The criteria for evaluating, categorizing, comparing, and predicting may become quite arbitrary and be inconsistent with what our *direct* experience (that is, sensory and present-moment experience) would tell us. For example, learning that making mistakes is bad can lead us to constrict our search for new solutions to problems, and to duck in an effort to go unnoticed by those we fear would criticize us, when, in fact, exploring and making *more* mistakes that we *notice* would serve us better.

As humans, we are continually invited to suffer. It is a distinction of dubious value to be the only species that can take a positive event, imbue it with negative qualities, and turn it into an opportunity to suffer. For example, imagine that you are on the vacation of a lifetime with good friends. You are looking at the ocean and having a great conversation with them. Maybe you are eating your favorite foods, too, and the sunset is beautiful— *but* your mind thinks, *If only my brother (sister, mom, or dad) could have lived to see this.* Bam! There it is—pain, the pain of living and losing someone, and perhaps suffering will come along too. For example, you might struggle to avoid immediately experiencing the thought and feeling; go back to your room, eliminating the possibility of connecting with others; or drink too much alcohol in order to numb out (Törneke & Luoma, 2009). Suffering becomes pervasive in our lives when we organize our behavior around controlling or avoiding the natural, clean pain life has in store for us. Again, this is something you see every day in medical practice: the patient who uses drugs to avoid memories of past trauma, the patient who settles for a life of being spaced out on pain medication to get away from back pain, the patient who overeats to compensate for feeling lonely, and so on.

When the control or elimination of personal pain becomes our focus, we lose sight of what's important for living a vital, purposeful life. This is what we call *psychological rigidity*. Lacking the skills we need to flexibly experience the pain, we continue to execute avoidance-based strategies to avoid or control suffering, and as our rigidity grows, so does our suffering, which is how we "get stuck." The alternative, *psychological flexibility*, is learning to be aware and accepting of the pain that comes into our lives while continuing to pursue what we value.

THE PRINCIPLE OF DESTRUCTIVE NORMALITY

Now, we will look systematically at suffering from an elements-of-mental-activity framework. Human beings do not behave randomly when confronted with some type of painful circumstance. From childhood, we are trained to address personal pain in a particular way. Early on, we learn that negative emotions need to be eliminated or, at worst, controlled, not because they are harmful, but because they have an emotional impact on others. The main reason we want a patient to stop crying in the exam room (apart from our fear of running late) is that crying makes us uncomfortable. We feel compelled to do something to "help the patient feel better" (such as stop the crying). Culturally this programming results in a hugely destructive social myth we call the *principle of destructive normality*: healthy people do not have negative mental experiences (particularly ones that they express to others), or if they do, they can control them as they arise. From a mechanistic perspective, we may unwittingly try to help our patients meet the cultural expectation of what's normal, encouraging our patients to control or reduce mental experiences.

The idea that feeling bad is bad for you is often paired with another cultural rule consistent with a mechanistic perspective: to figure out how to stop feeling bad, you need to figure out what's causing those feelings (for example, negative thoughts, traumatic memories, personal history) and eliminate the cause. Individuals who follow these rules are headed for suffering because of two scientific truths:

- Multiple studies have shown that attempts to suppress, control, or eliminate negative emotions, thoughts, memories, or sensations create a "rebound" effect that's associated with high levels of distress (Wegner, Schneider, Carter, & White, 1987).

- Humans bring their entire learning history into each moment, and this learning cannot be undone. It's impossible to control or eliminate your own history. The human nervous system only goes in one direction: forward from here. Memories cannot be erased, negative thoughts cannot be unlearned, and conditioned emotional reactions cannot be eliminated.

TEAMS: A FRAMEWORK FOR EXPLORING A CONTEXTUAL APPROACH TO SUFFERING

We offer the TEAMS acronym to help you develop a contextual perspective toward key elements of mental activity, including "T" for thoughts, "E" for emotions, "A" for associations, "M" for memories, and "S" for sensations. We will briefly explore the use of two metaphors, mind as a machine and mind as context, to clarify differences between mechanistic and contextual approaches, then introduce you to a contextual approach to each TEAMS element. Please heed this note of caution: we are not suggesting that mechanism is wrong and contextualism is right. We are asking that you add ACT, as a contextual approach to suffering, to your efforts to care for your patients. We believe this change will pay dividends right away!

Mind-as-a-Machine Model. This method suggests using direct control strategies to reduce symptoms of suffering. Our motives are compassionate, and at the same time, our strategy is very systematic. We approach the mind as we might approach a computer, removing problem-causing software (or negative thoughts) or adding more memory (or inhibiting serotonin reuptake). This approach encourages us to follow treatment rules and, combined with the pressure of time-limited visits, may make us less sensitive to our direct experience with patients and less flexible in our approach. For example, we might be puzzled by a patient's difficulties with increasing her positive thoughts or by reported nonimprovement in response to a therapeutic dose of an antidepressant. The mechanistic perspective would suggest that there's a reason for these unexpected results, and we might settle on a reason that does little to further our treatment. For example, the patient who does not improve his frequency of positive thoughts might be seen as "dysthymic" or "not trying," and the patient who is not responding to antidepressants might be seen as "treatment resistant" or "needing an augmentation medicine."

Mind-as-Context Model. Three elements of contextual theory are important in working with patients:

■ What is "true" is defined by *what works* for the patient. This means that there's no single path that people must follow to live healthy and fulfilling lives; negative thoughts do not need to diminish and medication does not need to alleviate symptoms before we begin pursuing a better life.

■ You cannot separate the patient from the two main contexts the patient is interacting with: the external environment and the internal environment—the world "between the ears." Both of these contexts interact with and exert an influence over the patient. With respect to the world between the ears, we liken the mind to a bowl of soup with many ingredients. Each ingredient has its context, including its history and the extent to which it impacts a person's functioning at the moment. It's possible for the human to carry this bowl rather than be carried by it, and when the human carries the bowl of mental content, new choices about behavior in the world are not only possible; they are probable.

■ As another person in the exam room, you are participating in the patient's external and internal contexts, and the patient is participating in yours. One saying we often use is, "There are really four of us in here today: you, me, your mind, and my mind!"

Now, we will look at each TEAMS element—thoughts, emotions, associations, memories, and sensations—from a contextual perspective.

Thoughts

Thoughts begin early in life, with the beginning of language acquisition. Very young, preverbal children cannot use words and have very restricted symbolic abilities. The acquisition of words and their meanings, taught first by parents, derives initially from associations with objects: "This is a dog; say 'dog.' What is this?" asks the parent while pointing to a picture of a dog. The parent prompts further, "Say 'dog'; how do you spell 'dog'?" reinforcing our ability to learn the sound, pictorial representation, and spelling, as well as how to categorize ("four-legged creatures" or "pets") and evaluate ("A dog is a man's best friend" or "Dogs are dangerous"). Our capacity to form relationships among stimuli expands rapidly, and soon we begin to apply this ability to form arbitrary or indirectly trained relations; for example, "Dogs are dangerous, so dog owners cannot be trusted." Soon in some contexts, strings of words come to exert more influence over our behavior than our direct experience in those contexts, because we learn to see the world through language: we partition some things, categorize other things; evaluate and compare, predict and forecast. All of these operations occur at the level of thought, and because it's an ongoing process, we tend to get very "cozy" with our "word machine."

From a conceptual perspective, we understand that patients may not be aware of their thoughts as thoughts and rules about life, and we do not assume that they need to change their thoughts to improve their lives. We attempt to help patients become more present and aware of their thoughts as thoughts (rather than *truths* with a capital "T"). We also support their efforts to develop the skills necessary to take action in ways that work in their life contexts. For example, we might encourage a frustrated parent of a child with ADHD to be aware of and accepting of thoughts like "I'm not a good parent," while delivering an effective behavioral response to the child (such as touch the child's shoulder, ask for eye contact, make a specific request, and then ask the child to repeat it). With ongoing support from a PCP using a contextual perspective, patients can improve their skills at working with their thoughts, using them when they work in their life contexts and just "holding" them with compassion when they don't.

Emotions

The Latin root of the word "emotion" literally means "movement." Functioning to motivate behavior, emotions are known to be present from the first moments of life. They create both positive (such as happiness) and negative (such as sadness or anger) internal states. Like thoughts, they come and go moment to moment most of our lives.

While emotions appear to be our birthright and to have survival value, our cultural training can make it threatening to experience emotions directly. Lacking adequate information about emotions, our parents and teachers may be unable to model acceptance of emotions and, instead, insist on control: "Stop crying, or I'll give you something to cry about!" "Why can't you just be happy, like me!" Since, as children, we cannot directly observe how well our models suppress or control their emotions, most of us infer from the language they use that they are much more successful than we are. And from about age seven, we secretly suspect that there's something wrong with us, that our emotions are somehow defective. Our culture reifies rational, deductive reasoning and views intuition, inspiration, emotions, and similar nonverbal experiences with suspicion.

The irony is that emotions are never wrong; they have evolved over the aeons to become our most basic "signaling system." Emotions tell us something very important about the immediate world and whether it's working toward our best interests. It is our language-shaped processes that create suffering, because we are taught to ignore our signaling system. *Emotional intelligence* (EI) is the extent to which we are able to engage in value-consistent behavior in the context of difficult emotions and emotionally charged thoughts (Ciarrochi, Forgas, & Mayer, 2006; Ciarrochi & Mayer, 2007). Primary care providers can play a central role in emotional intelligence training by focusing less on the patient's verbal reasoning and more on the patient's acceptance of emotional experience and ability to behave in value-consistent ways. For purposes of illustration, consider an adolescent patient who seeks help because her head hurts but then explains that she is angry with her parents because they continue to treat her "like a child." Her experience of anger is providing her with a signal, and the PCP can help her pay attention to this signal and use it to initiate a behavior that will work better for her (for example, she might discuss her curfew and telephone and computer time limits with her parents rather than resort to throwing temper tantrums).

Associations

Associations are mental operations that link experiences sharing common properties—often connecting something that is happening now (such as a thought, emotion, or sensation) to something that happened before (such as a memory)—and frame how we organize and use mental elements (for example, rules we have learned from models, such as *Make good grades and you'll have a good life*, or rules we have derived from experience, such as *Don't tell people you're afraid, or they'll think you're incompetent*).

Very early in life, we learn to *frame* our experience. For example, we learn a frame for comparing, and we apply it to our external environment (*This chair is larger than that chair*) and our internal environment (*I feel worse today than I did yesterday* or *She's smarter than I am*). We also have frames that lead us to look at similarities and differences, for example, with reference to other professionals (*I'm a doctor, and you are a nurse*), ethnic or religious groups, or community groups (*I'm a Republican, and you are too*). We combine frames, and this ability helps us solve some problems but causes others, such as stigmata, prejudices, and stereotypes.

Associations and frames can evoke powerful responses in a positive or negative direction; for example, a citizen may feel a strong sense of patriotism when hearing his national anthem. In clinical practice, a patient with a somatic focus who frames you as "just the same as all those other doctors who won't take the time to figure out what's causing my dizziness and aches and pains" can evoke frustration, which, whether spoken or unspoken, impacts care. From a contextual point of view, associations function as "triggers" for specific thoughts, emotions, memories, sensations, and behaviors, as well as organizers or frames for our mental events.

Try thinking of associations as thickeners in our mind-as-a-bowl-of-soup metaphor. They bind things together using words that suggest relationships, such as "if..., then"; "now..., then"; "better..., worse"; and "I..., you." Our ability to make associations or place frames on our perspective underlies our gift for generating behaviors based on rules. Once associations become linked to certain events, it's impossible to reverse the association. The appearance of a learned association cannot be eradicated; it can only be accepted. For example, a soldier returning from a war zone where roadside bombs were commonplace can learn to accept, but cannot "delete," the experience of fear when seeing a bag of trash on the side of a road. A patient who has formed a frame or rule like *If I have pain, the doctor should give me something to stop it* can add to that rule (*Maybe the doctor can help me better manage my pain*) but not delete it. Some rules help us (for example, *Don't walk through an intersection on a red light, or you'll get hurt*), and some get us stuck in living out losing story lines about our lives (for example, *Mistakes are bad, and I have made so many that I'll never amount to anything*).

Memories

Memories are mental operations that allow us to bring forward elements of our past experiences. They often trigger associations with a wide range of thoughts, feelings, and sensations. As we recall an event, we may come to reexperience parts of it, even though it is long past. From a contextual point of view, humans naturally experience memories in many forms (such as stories, pictures, and smells), both consciously and unconsciously, and when memories are painful, the tendency is to avoid thinking about them and to avoid situations that might trigger them. For example, the war veteran may close the curtains to avoid seeing cars that evoke memories of roadside bomb explosions. However, these memories were already present when the curtains were closed, and they may actually become more intrusive when avoided. Further, the drawn curtains close off the possibility of witnessing a more life-affirming experience, such as a friendly exchange between two people meeting on the street. It is the avoidance of memories, not the memories themselves, that produces the toxic effect.

Sensations

While "sensations" comes last in our TEAMS acronym, it usually comes first when our patients come to see us in primary care. Sensations include each of the five senses separately and in various combinations. During medical visits, we may hear patients spontaneously describe sensory experiences, such as "My back feels like it is on fire" or "My head is pounding." Sensations are also the somatic results of mental activity, as with the depressed patient who complains of headache, fatigue, or belly pain. Of course, we use our senses in our practice of medicine: "This lump feels hard and mobile," or "This ear seems to be occluded with wax."

Sensations are interesting ingredients in the bowl, because they occur in the present moment. An endless array of beats and gurgles and tickles is happening in the human body at any given time. It is our language that directs our attention to these sensations and then ascribes meaning to them. In the contextual approach, sensations become problematic when we evaluate them in highly provocative ways: *My heart is beating fast. This isn't right. There must be something wrong, possibly a heart attack. My father died of a heart attack. I need to get to a doctor.* Sensations are also a problem when we begin to use self-defeating strategies designed to avoid them: *I need a really stiff drink to get rid of my anxiety.* Sensations and our evaluations of them may trigger use of necessary and unnecessary medical services. Often, patients present worrisome sensations as a "ticket" for entrance to primary care. Primary care providers are well positioned to help patients tune in to sensations and use them to anchor their attention to the here and now.

WHAT DOES ACT BRING TO THE BEHAVIOR-CHANGE AGENDA?

As a contextual approach to psychological suffering, ACT attempts not to cure patients of their symptoms, but to improve their ability to consistently pursue meaningful lives, whatever their life challenges—physical, mental, or both. While a new approach, ACT is a contextual approach that's now associated with improving care for diabetes patients (Gregg, Callaghan, Hayes, & Glenn-Lawson, 2007); patients who smoke (Gifford et al., 2004); patients with chronic pain (McCracken & Eccleston, 2003; Dahl et al., 2004); patients with uncontrolled seizure disorder (Lundgren et al., 2008); and patients with mental health problems commonly treated in the primary care setting, including depression (Zettle & Rains, 1989), opiate addiction maintained with methadone (Hayes, Wilson, et al., 2004), and anxiety (Hayes et al., 2006). ACT teaches patients to acknowledge and accept the appearance of distressing TEAMS, to clarify what would be a value-based response to these unwanted experiences, and to take effective action in that direction. Rather than support the cultural model that the "good life" is being symptom free, ACT suggests that PCPs normalize the role of symptoms of psychological distress in the human life and teach patients to attend to symptoms as signals while moving forward in life. As a PCP, you are well positioned to deliver this powerful and healing message to your patients so that over the long haul, they are better able to live meaningful lives.

SUMMARY

Since we covered a lot of territory in our first chapter, let's review the basics:

- Given a lack of continued improvement in outcomes produced by cognitive behavioral therapy, psychologists have explored new strategies for changing behavior.

- Relational frame theory offers a behavioral analytic model of human language.

- While the biomedical approach suggests that we look at the "form" of a patient's complaints and symptoms, a contextual approach asks us to look at the function of the symptoms or the way the symptoms impact the patient's life.

■ The contextual approach encourages us to look at the interaction a patient has with internal (mental) and external (environmental) contexts.

■ Pain, a normal part of life, differs from suffering, which we might think of as additional pain and struggle originating in our ability to evaluate, categorize, compare, and predict.

■ The principle of destructive normality is a part of our cultural programming that suggests that healthy people do not have negative mental experiences or, if they do, they are able to control them.

■ The TEAMS (thoughts, emotions, associations, memories, sensations) acronym helps you attend to the key elements of mental activity, the patient's as well as your own.

■ Think of the mind as a context rather than a machine, and you'll be set to learn and use new techniques for creating real behavior change in your patients and in your practice.

■ This book provides you with a new tool kit for creating real behavior change, based on acceptance and commitment therapy (ACT). ACT takes a contextual approach to psychological suffering and suggests that you not attempt to cure patients of their symptoms, but help them improve their ability to consistently pursue meaningful lives, whatever their life challenges—physical, mental, or both.

PREVIEW

Chapter 2 provides information about six core processes that contribute to psychological inflexibility and suffering (Six Core Processes: Psychological Rigidity), and chapter 3 introduces six core processes that may promote psychological flexibility and vitality (Six Core Processes: Psychological Flexibility). Chapter 4, the last chapter in the first part of the book, introduces you to a variety of tools to use in creating real behavior change.

CHAPTER 2

How People Get Stuck

For a long time, it had seemed to me that life was about to begin—
real life. But there was always some obstacle in the way, something to
be gotten through first, some unfinished business, time still to be served,
a debt to be paid. Then life would begin. At last it dawned on me that
these obstacles were my life.

—Alfred D. Souza

The contextual approach suggests that patients get stuck when they behave as if they *are* the ingredients of the "soup" rather than the bowl that *holds* them. Statements like "I'm a smoker and I'll always be one" and "My heart attack has ruined any chance I have of living a good life" reveal that the patient's identity is defined by a specific thought, evaluation, and emotion. Overidentifying with the content of TEAMS leads to behavior patterns that don't respond to real-world "inputs," a state we refer to as *psychological rigidity*. Psychologically rigid individuals are prone to suffering and maladaptive behavior, because their negative TEAMS function as barriers to vital living. They take their TEAMS as literal truth and can't distinguish themselves from the content of their experiences between the ears. In this chapter, we will introduce you to the key elements of psychological rigidity. When you understand the six processes that trap your patients in unworkable patterns of behavior, you will be in a better position to help them develop the psychological flexibility they need to address the life challenges they are facing and to bring more meaning to their lives.

SIX CORE PROCESSES: PSYCHOLOGICAL RIGIDITY

How can a person use ineffective methods to control suffering for years and not figure out a way to change things? How can an intelligent, caring person do the same unworkable thing over and over again? How can a person live a life that's disconnected from his personal values? These are the questions that come up when you see a patient with COPD who continues to smoke, a patient with alcohol dependence who continues to drink despite severe health consequences, a patient with chronic back pain who withdraws from life in an attempt to control pain. In this section, we will answer these questions by describing six mental processes that collectively cause people to stay stuck for months, years, and even a lifetime.

As you recall from chapter 1, human behavior is organized through language and thinking, and we learn to follow rules and engage in rule-governed behavior.

Our learning context can be characterized as predominantly appetitive or aversive. When our behavior is under *appetitive control*, it is geared toward receiving positive reinforcement and tends to be flexible and exploratory, producing desirable consequences. When our behavior is under *aversive control*, it is designed to help us avoid or escape from aversive stimulation, and it tends to be rigid, rule bound, and generally avoidant.

When people grow up in families where aversive control is the paradigm, they tend to suffer a great deal as adults and to have difficulty making behavior changes and solving problems. Most of us are governed by appetitive control in some areas of our lives and by aversive control in other areas. As the number of our areas that are under aversive control grows, we are more likely to demonstrate unworkable patterns of coping behavior.

Figure 2.1 pictorially represents the six psychological mechanisms that contribute to psychological rigidity. While patients typically are stronger in some areas and weaker in others, these processes are highly related, and significant problems in one area often contribute to problems in one or more other areas. We will describe each of these life-robbing processes, beginning at the twelve o'clock position and working clockwise around the hexagon depicting the core processes that contribute to psychological rigidity.

FIGURE 2.1
Six Core Processes: Psychological Rigidity

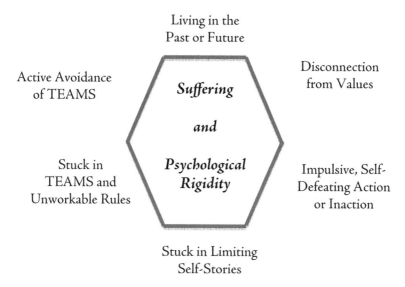

Living in the
Past or Future

Active Avoidance
of TEAMS

Suffering

and

Disconnection
from Values

Stuck in
TEAMS and
Unworkable Rules

*Psychological
Rigidity*

Impulsive, Self-
Defeating Action
or Inaction

Stuck in Limiting
Self-Stories

Living in the Past or Future

From an ACT point of view, psychological rigidity develops when the patient has trouble being "present" and tends to spend mental life in the past or future. Human minds are not built to "be here now," because there's very little role for symbolic activity in the now. For example, by the time you describe what you are thinking, you are thinking something else. The "now" is ahead of language and symbolic activity. In a very basic way, patients who ruminate incessantly over unfair things that have happened to them are going to spend a lot of emotional energy dealing with sadness, grief, guilt, and anger. Typically, patients with multiple symptoms of depression are vulnerable to allowing the past to dominate their present-moment experience. Patients who live in the future will be faced with apprehension, worry, and anxiety. It's interesting to note that most positive emotions are "right here, right now" experiences, whereas negative emotions tend to have a past or future focus.

Disconnection from Values

When patients are disconnected from their values, they are unable to use them to guide their actions. Instead, patients will follow socially inculcated rules that substitute for personally meaningful, chosen life goals. In ACT, we call these rules *plys*, and a pattern of rule following is called *pliance*. For example, the straight-A college student might want to "please" her parents by becoming a dentist, because her parents cherish the status of having a "doctor" in the family (a ply). Consequently, the student avoids pursuing her dream of becoming a teacher, even though she doesn't really expect dentistry to be a fulfilling career (pliance). Patients with learning histories heavily based in pliance can easily lose sight of what they want their lives to be about, particularly if they are immersed in complicated life situations they can't manage by following overly general rules. For many patients with chronic pain, even if their pain miraculously disappeared, they wouldn't know where to go with life. Similarly, a patient struggling with depression may tell his doctor, "I have a job, a family, even a nice car—and I'm still unhappy." Unfortunately, simply having a family, a job, and a nice car is not a formula for happiness; it is a social myth. In ACT, we talk about the experience of climbing a ladder and finding out at the top that it's up against the wrong wall. In other words, we can engage in sustained goal-directed behavior based on rules about how to live, and in the end feel that our lives are shallow and devoid of meaning. The problem of burnout in the medical professions is an excellent example of this type of process.

Impulsive, Self-Defeating Action or Inaction

Psychological rigidity is characterized by ineffective behaviors like impulsive or self-defeating actions, such as avoidance and withdrawal, or both. Passivity, or inaction, involves not engaging in needed behaviors, and it may be due to behavior-skill deficits (for example, lack of effective assertion skills or problem-solving skills). This occurs when a patient avoids events, situations, or interactions that though potentially unpleasant, need to be approached and resolved in some way. Behavioral avoidance eliminates the possibility of positive reinforcement but increases the possibility of negative reinforcement. For example, a depressed patient who avoids a social gathering due to low energy will feel more depressed and have even less energy afterward. What is sacrificed is the possibility of meeting someone at the gathering who would be supportive of the patient. Behavioral excesses are actions that, though used frequently, are self-defeating. Not surprisingly, these behaviors generate a vast amount of negative life outcomes and associated negative TEAMS. Behaviors like binge drinking, drugging, and over-eating only add fuel to the negative TEAMS fire. Large groups of patients struggling to make needed changes so they can better self-manage chronic disease likely have deficits in this area.

Stuck in Limiting Self-Stories

The self-story is the way you describe who you are and how you came to be that way. Self-stories can support workable behavior or perpetuate patterns of unworkable behavior. *Low perspective taking* means that a person cannot see that he is telling a story. In other words, the story is the only reality. *High perspective taking* is being able to see that you are telling a story, and that the story could and does change. With high-perspective-taking ability, a person can see storytelling as a process and let the story be just a story rather than the ultimate truth.

Everyone has a self-story, and what it contains varies according to the context. Consider the difference between your response to "Tell me about yourself" at a job interview and your response during a medical visit. The aspects of the self-story someone might produce at a job interview would tend to highlight why the interviewer might want to hire that person. During an initial medical visit, a new patient typically provides a brief statement about her health history and current health concerns. What we are most concerned about is self-stories that function as a sort of self-fulfilling prophecy; for example, the patient with uncontrolled diabetes who states, "I've never really succeeded at anything that was important to me in my life. I just seem to sabotage myself. This will probably be just another one of those times when I fail at something that's really important." The patient who identifies with the self-story as being literally true sets the stage for rigid behavior patterns and resultant suffering. The point here is that the self-story is a product of language and, at some level, is an arbitrary collection of remembered experiences and imputed cause-and-effect relationships. Scientifically speaking, no self-story is accurate, because millions of elements of personal learning history are either left out or are not consciously accessible.

From an ACT point of view, having a self-story is not a problem in and of itself. The problem is holding the self-story as if it were true, particularly when the story focuses on negative life outcomes in the past and predicts similar outcomes in the future. Holding a story in this way suggests low-perspective-taking ability. Another suggestion of limited perspective-taking skills is when a patient provides a self-story to justify why he can't change or ever be different in any substantive way. These self-stories function more as a social justification for why the patient will never succeed at anything important. This type of story quells motivation to even begin to try something different and is very frustrating for medical providers. Even a positive self-story (for example, "I am strong and don't need any help") can lead to problems (such as refusal to use medications for a medical problem) when held inflexibly and without the skill of shifting perspectives on the story. In ACT, we often say that the most dangerous aspect of human language is the "conceptualized self" that appears in our self-story. Even though this version of self-knowledge may cause enormous suffering, patients defend the story as if their lives depended on it.

Stuck in TEAMS and Unworkable Rules

A word that describes the extent to which humans can get stuck in TEAMS and unworkable rules is "fusion." *Mental fusion* is consistently overidentifying with the content of private experience (such as TEAMS). The Latin root of the word "fusion" literally means "to be poured together." In this case, the patient is poured together with one or more TEAMS elements. It is quite common in medical visits to see the lack of space between the patient, as a person, and the thing with which he is fused. As an example, consider the patient with symptoms of panic who insists, "I'm afraid that something's wrong with my heart and that I'm going to die from a heart attack. I need to go to the ER right now!" In this moment of fusion, the patient's ability to step back and see thoughts as thoughts, sensations as sensations, and emotions as emotions is severely limited. Fusion is not always bad; for example, when you cross a busy intersection, you need to immediately fuse with what your mind tells you to do. But in stressful or emotionally challenging situations, even a little space between TEAMS and the person experiencing TEAMS will reduce reflexive avoidance behaviors, stop ineffective rule following, and allow the person to respond more effectively.

Active Avoidance of TEAMS

Experiential avoidance is the unwillingness to make contact with distressing, unwanted private experiences (TEAMS), and it typically involves avoidance, suppression, distraction, and escape. This process has been repeatedly shown in studies to be a root cause of almost every known form of psychopathology (Hayes, Wilson, Gifford, Follette, & Strosahl, 1996). Along with mental fusion, avoidance is the very bedrock of psychological rigidity. As is true of fusion, we all engage in experiential avoidance. Why? Remember our discussion of how we are dominated by language. We all have learned, and routinely apply, language rules related to problem solving. In reality, these rules work quite well with problems in the external world. The rules of problem solving include (1) identify a problem, (2) identify its cause, and (3) get rid of the cause, thereby eliminating the original problem. For example, (1) Jill has a sore throat, and (2) her streptococcal screen is positive, so (3) you prescribe antibiotics to kill the streptococci, thereby ridding her of the sore throat.

Unfortunately, when we apply these three easy steps to the problem of negative TEAMS, the problem gets bigger, not better. Let's take the problem of compassion fatigue. A provider might look inside herself and decide that the cause is "not being strong enough" and the solution is to "exert better emotional control" (suppression), thereby eliminating the original cause and, hopefully, the fatigue. Unfortunately, this strategy doesn't work over the long term. Eventually the provider will experience breakthrough compassion fatigue, feel a loss of emotional control, and possibly easily engage in internal (daydreaming, overcompensating) or external (calling in sick, or transferring or discharging "needy" patients) avoidance behaviors.

Basically, the less you want a certain thought, memory, emotion, or physical sensation, the more you will get of it. In ACT, we call this the "rule of mental events." As we mentioned in chapter 1, conscious attempts to suppress TEAMS elements lead to a paradoxical rebound effect and more emotional distress associated with the uncontrolled TEAMS. Interestingly, the paradoxical result of experiential avoidance is not readily apparent to most patients who are suffering. It usually requires specific questioning to uncover the real results the patient is getting from his emotional avoidance strategies (for example, "So, do you think exerting more control over your emotions has made your compassion fatigue better, or have you noticed that, strangely, it's getting worse?").

SUMMARY

In this chapter, you've learned about how people get stuck. Let's review the key ideas:

- Remember to tell your patients—and yourself—"Pain is inevitable; suffering is optional." Suffering grows when we struggle with the inevitable experience of pain in our daily lives.

- Our learning history can be considered as predominantly appetitive or aversive.

- Under appetitive control, our behavior is focused on receiving positive reinforcement and tends to be flexible and exploratory, producing desirable results.

- Under aversive control, our behavior helps us avoid or escape aversive stimulation and tends to be rigid, rule bound, and generally avoidant.

- Most of us are governed by appetitive control in some life areas and by aversive control in other areas. As our number of life areas under aversive control grows, we are more likely to display unworkable patterns of coping behavior.

- Rules learned under aversive-control conditions tend to be rigid, making it difficult for us to behave in ways inconsistent with the rules—or to even see that our experience doesn't fit with what a rule says.

- The more energy we expend on avoiding distressing TEAMS or real-world situations, the less energy we have for pursuing meaningful lives.

- The six core processes of psychological rigidity are 1) living in the past or future; 2) disconnecting from values; 3) impulsive, self-defeating action or inaction; 4) being stuck in limiting self-stories; 5) being stuck in TEAMS and unworkable rules; and 6) actively avoiding TEAMS.

- These life-robbing processes are the result of social conditioning.

As primary care providers, we can function as role models for how to escape the rigidity trap and move toward greater flexibility. We can do this by seeing the private experiences of our patients (and ourselves) for what they are: just ingredients in a bowl of soup. If we can remember that we are the bowls that contain the soup, we can teach patients to do the same in pursuit of important life outcomes. To do so, we need to look at our patients' suffering with "soft eyes" and realize, "There, but for the grace of God, go I."

PREVIEW

In chapter 3, we will introduce you to three very important real behavior change concepts: workability, values, and vital living. We will also examine six distinct processes that contribute to psychological flexibility and vitality (Six Core Processes: Psychological Flexibility).

CHAPTER 3

Creating a Context for Change

When the music changes, so does the dance.

—African proverb

The music in our lives includes our TEAMS, our behavioral responses to them, and the difficult psychosocial stressors we experience from time to time in our families, relationships, work, and community. This dance, at any given moment, can move us toward either suffering or vitality. When patients get stuck, you, the health care professional, are often the first person they see, so you are in an excellent position to "redefine" the problem in contextual terms and help them shift from processes that promote psychological rigidity to those that promote psychological flexibility.

In this chapter, we will introduce a simple but elegant intervention model you can use to address sources of psychological rigidity and the resultant suffering of your patients. First, we will examine two very important concepts: how patients who are stuck tend to focus their energies on things they can't change (TEAMS), resulting in a loss of focus on things they *can* change (daily actions); and using the notion of "workability" to undermine this negative process and help them shift their focus back to controllable outcomes. This "prelude" is often necessary to get patients into a mind-set in which change seems possible and resistance to new ideas is lessened. We will then discuss six ACT processes that will function as antidotes to the rigidity-producing processes we outlined in the previous chapter. We will present specific techniques you can use to activate the six core processes of psychological flexibility. You can use these techniques in ten-minute consultations with patients. By applying these procedures, you can help patients improve their physical and emotional health, even when life circumstances are difficult and TEAMS are unpleasant.

> Remember, when this symbol appears next to discussions about a diagram or worksheet, you can find a copy online at http://www .newharbingeronline.com/real-behavior-change-in-primary-care.html.

DETECTING AND UNDERMINING THE UNWORKABLE BEHAVIOR-CHANGE AGENDA

Ultimately, the goal of any primary care intervention is to get the patient to change behavior. We often joke that medicine is 10 percent technical knowledge and 90 percent behavior-change skills. Even a medical instruction as innocuous as asking a patient to take a medication will trigger forces in her internal context (attitudes, beliefs, expectations, and other potentially difficult TEAMS) and external context that will determine the eventual form of any behavior change or whether a change will occur at all. We have seen many a situation in which a family member "convinced" a patient not to take a needed medicine because of issues the family member had with using drugs to treat even a bona fide medical problem. Thus, it's important to pay attention to how internal and external contexts influence the results of your behavior-change discussions with the patient.

Reason Giving

When patients fail to distinguish between internal and external contexts, they tend to apply strategies that work in the external world to internal problems, and they rely on the insidious process of reason giving. Reasons can function as justifications for and explanations of problematic behaviors. For example, one patient with diabetes "explains" that his out-of-control hemoglobin A1c is due to a broken glucometer. Another patient explains that it's because she is depressed, and once she gets rid of the depression, she will be able to control her diabetes better. The purpose is to give you a plausible explanation of what's going on, such that you will be, at least, *somewhat* sympathetic, and to present you with a problem to solve so that the diabetes is more amenable to control. The reason behind "fixing the glucometer" is external, and the behavior-change solution is doable and observable and may help with diabetes control. But getting rid of the depression first is a strategy that won't work for dealing with a group of private, distressing TEAMS, and this approach won't likely improve control of the patient's diabetes.

Reasons figure prominently in stories patients tell about themselves, and reasons exert an important social function in interactions between patients and PCPs. Less-flexible patients often reason that effective action is impossible when distressing TEAMS are present, and they ask their PCPs to help them control or eliminate distressing TEAMS *before* they begin to act in more value-consistent ways. Unfortunately, neither the PCP nor the patient can wave distressing TEAMS away, and in fact trying to suppress or control them may make them worse.

A Lack of Cultural Instruction

The problem is that there's very little cultural instruction in what to do about distressing TEAMS, so most patients simply extrapolate from how they solve problems in the external world. They are "trapped" in following the only approach they know to address the problem of how to live a vital life. In ACT, we call this conundrum the *unworkable change agenda*. To have any chance of really helping your patient, you must first undermine the change agenda the patient has been following, and in a way that doesn't create resistance or drive a wedge into your relationship.

WORKABILITY: THE CATALYST FOR CHANGE

Workability is a key term in creating a context for behavior change. A workable life is one that is producing desired outcomes on an ongoing basis. Your job is to help the patient live a life that produces outcomes that matter to that person. To catalyze change, we need to understand patients' motives for living and whether their behaviors are moving them in the direction of those motives. With few exceptions, humans are interested in living lives that allow them to laugh, love, and experience joy. They want to feel "useful" in their daily lives, to have fulfilling relationships, and to smell the roses of life. This is far easier said than done in most everyone's life. Most individuals earn workability by addressing myriad life challenges that unfold sequentially over a life span. As one famous old saying in therapy goes: "Life is one darned thing after another. Your job is to make sure it's not the *same* darned thing!"

To assess workability during a patient encounter, you will need to ask about four domains: motive, behavior, short-term results, and long-term results (see sample worksheet 3.1). Try practicing these questions with a patient or in a practice session with a colleague. Sample worksheet 3.1 provides an example of a person with COPD who is experiencing frequent anxiety attacks triggered by chest tightness and shortness of breath that's at least partly related to the disease process. Often, avoidance-based strategies (as we discussed in chapter 2) produce desirable short-term consequences (because they relieve or prevent aversive TEAMS) but have devastating long-term consequences. In contrast, *approach-oriented strategies* can, and often do, generate distressing TEAMS in the short run, but if the patient doesn't revert back to avoidance, the long-term consequences are much more in line with the patient's best interests. Nearly always, patients who are stuck and suffering are making the trade-off of gaining immediate relief from distressing TEAMS in exchange for sacrificing their long-term best interests. To create real behavior change, we help the patient listen to herself when she answers the questions about motive, behavior, short-term results, and long-term results.

SAMPLE WORKSHEET 3.1
COPD Patient's Workability Analysis

Motive	Behavior	Short-Term Results	Long-Term Results
What outcomes are you trying to achieve? What outcomes are most important to you (best serve your interests)?	*What are you doing?*	*What happens in the short term?*	*What happens in the long run?*
Avoidance-Based Strategies			
Avoid distressing TEAMS triggered by COPD symptoms and associated anxiety	Rest at home, avoid exerting myself	Fewer episodes of chest tightness, less anxiety about dying	Loss of participation in family activities, isolation from friends and social connections
Control exposure to stress-producing situations that create symptoms	Appease spouse and friends during disagreements, remove self from interaction rather than assert self	Reduced stress and associated fearful chest symptoms, less anxiety about dying	Resentment about giving in to pressure, not getting needs met; loss of real connection with spouse, friends; feelings of isolation
Approach-Oriented Strategies			
Participate in important life activities and learn to live with physical COPD symptoms	Engage spouse and friends directly, express opinions and needs, stay in stressful situations even though physical symptoms are present	Initial higher likelihood of chest symptoms and anxious thoughts, possibility of having an outright anxiety attack	Increased sense of intimacy and connection with spouse and friends, improved self-image, feelings of well-being associated with getting social needs met

In practice, this patient might ask you for advice on how to better prevent or eliminate any chest symptoms in order to improve quality of life. In this case, after discussing the four elements of workability, the PCP might say, "So, I'm hearing that your main strategy has been to avoid any situation that might trigger the sensation of chest tightness and shortness of breath. It sounds as if you've done that very well and consistently, so I can tell you are able to stick with something if you think it will work. What I'm wondering is, *stepping back* and looking at how this approach has affected your life situation over time, do you feel that this strategy has been working? Do you feel that it's promoting the kind of life you are seeking in terms of your relationship with your spouse and friends, and how you get your needs met?" The workability question is the great equalizer in conversations about change. It forces the patient to look directly at results (a self-discovery of what is and isn't working) without requiring you to tell her what is and isn't working (which will raise resistance and increase the likelihood that the patient will continue using the unworkable strategy).

WORKABILITY, VITALITY, AND PSYCHOLOGICAL FLEXIBILITY

The ultimate goal of ACT is to help patients lead more vital and purposeful lives in the areas of life that matter to most patients (such as work, love, play, health, spirituality, and friendships). This means lives that are characterized by strength, skillfulness in taking an active and effective approach to problems of living, and sustained value-consistent action patterns. It does not mean a life free of disease or psychological distress. Disease is a part of aging; we all break down over time.

John Last (1988) suggests that health is a state of physical and psychological integrity with the ability to respond effectively to biopsychosocial stresses; optimal performance in family, work, and community roles; freedom from risk of disease and untimely death; and the experience of vitality. This definition emphasizes the patient's ability to respond and adapt, and it encourages a focus on the interconnectivity of human health with the health of other entities. Understanding the impact of avoidance-based problem solving will give you an opportunity to help patients move toward approach-oriented strategies. *Vitality*, the feeling of being "really" alive, is possible under all the dreadful and troubling life circumstances we experience, once we take an approach orientation, which requires skill at using the six core processes that support psychological flexibility.

SIX CORE PROCESSES: PSYCHOLOGICAL FLEXIBILITY

Psychological flexibility means being able to be present in the moment, fully aware and open to our experience, and to take action consistent with our values. More simply, it is stepping back from painful TEAMS and unworkable rules about life, and accepting them for what they are, focusing on the present, connecting with our larger sense of self, and moving toward what really matters to us. It's about acceptance, choice, and action! Six core processes support the ongoing ability to flexibly change our behavior and pursue vitality (see figure 3.1; additional copies of this figure are in appendix F and online). Now, we will begin at twelve o'clock on the hexagon and move in a clockwise direction, defining each of these processes and describing several techniques that activate them. Please note that while we present these processes separately for purposes of teaching, they are, of course, highly interrelated. Many patients benefit from work on a single process, because results from that work kindle growth in other processes. It's usually best to focus on a single process in a visit and to use one or two techniques to help the patient move toward a more meaningful life. In follow-up visits, you and your patient may continue with that process or go to a new one. Rather than follow a sequential protocol, select the process and technique needed to address the behavior-change needs of your patient at any particular point in time.

FIGURE 3.1 Six Core Processes: Psychological Flexibility

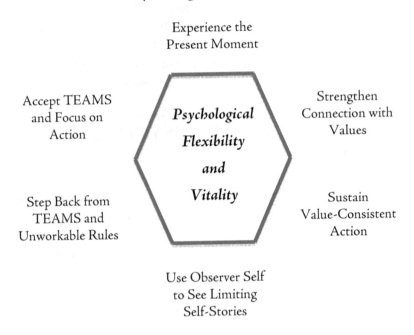

Experience the
Present Moment

Accept TEAMS
and Focus on
Action

Psychological

Flexibility

and

Vitality

Strengthen
Connection with
Values

Step Back from
TEAMS and
Unworkable Rules

Sustain
Value-Consistent
Action

Use Observer Self
to See Limiting
Self-Stories

Experience the Present Moment

This process involves the patient's ability to "be here now." Being in the present moment is not a strong suit of the human mind, for there's little need to think about being in the present moment when you are *in* the moment. Thinking about it immediately draws you *out* of the moment. So, the human mind's central strength resides in its ability to evaluate, categorize, and relate past events and experiences and to project past learning into analysis or prediction of the immediate and distant future. While these formidable abilities can enhance solutions to some problems, they can lead our patients to miss out on what's happening in the here-and-now moment in life so they can learn from that experience. Learning a few skills for entering the present moment offers patients relief from the problems of "there and then" and "what if" mind wars.

TECHNIQUES TO ENHANCE
PRESENT-MOMENT EXPERIENCE

Time Line. The Time Line is an experiential technique (often helpful to patients with depression and anxiety; see chapter 8 for more information on how you might use it). You draw a horizontal line on a piece of paper and label the left end "the past" and the right end "the future." In the middle of the line, write, "the present." Then, place your finger on the line and begin to model watching your thoughts, feelings, and sensations as they appear, and tracing where they are on the line. For example, you might say, "I'm having the sensation of touching the paper with my finger—that's the present. And now I'm noticing a grumbling in my stomach—this is now, too. But now I'm thinking about what I'll have for lunch" (moving your finger toward the right, or "the future," side of the line). Then, invite your patient to try it for a minute or two. This allows you to check his understanding. Ask the patient if he is willing to practice the exercise every morning for five minutes, advising that he will probably get lost in the future or past—where the mind likes to hang out—and that keeping a finger on the line will help him come back to the present, where feeling the paper is possible.

Three (or Five) Senses. The Three (or Five) Senses technique is also experiential (see chapter 8 for a case example concerning anxiety and depression). As PCP, ask your patient to name three (or five) things she sees, then three things she hears, and continue with the senses of smell, taste, and touch. At the end of the three-to-five-minute exercise, you can explain that the patient just spent three to five minutes in the present moment.

Balloon Breath. In this exercise, as PCP, you teach the patient to breathe in a relaxed manner from the diaphragm (see chapter 9 for a case example concerning trauma). The cycle of breathing should be slow, approximately four seconds on the outbreath with a one-second pause, then four seconds on the inbreath with a one-second pause before repeating the cycle. We like to have the patient use the image of a balloon in the abdomen that empties on exhalation and fills on inhalation. Once the patient is able to follow the breath using the balloon image, you can suggest switching to using the word "here" when emptying and "now" when filling. A next step is to have the patient focus on an object in the room and continue using the words "here" and "now." This technique can serve as the basis for later homework assignments involving its use while the patient engages in planned exposure (through imagination or in real life) to previously avoided situations and TEAMS.

Strengthen Connection with Values

Values are global abstract concepts that serve to motivate meaningful action. Most patients are willing to talk with medical providers about their values, and talking about values often deepens the relationship between the PCP and patient. Activities that enhance a patient's clarity regarding important values may rectify the suffering that comes with weakened connections to personal ideals. In the following exercise, we recommend interventions the PCP can use to help patients form a stronger bond with their important values. The first two techniques help the patient clarify values, and the third helps the patient determine discrepancy between current behaviors and valued directions.

The Bull's Eye Worksheet is often a core part of ongoing interactions between PCPs and patients. Two of the three bull's-eye intervention components (Value Identification and Value–Behavior Discrepancy) help the patient form a stronger connection with values, while the third component (Action Steps) provides a structure for sustaining value-consistent action over time. You can use any one or all of the intervention components in a visit with a patient, depending on your time and the patient's readiness. Chapter 5 provides a case example that demonstrates all three components of the bull's-eye, and a variety of other chapters demonstrate individual components. In many other chapters, we focus on one or two components, and when we do, we refer to the Bull's-Eye Worksheet to indicate that the PCP is using one or more of its components.

TECHNIQUES TO STRENGTHEN
CONNECTION WITH VALUES

Retirement Party/Tombstone. This exercise is useful for PCPs and medical trainees, as well as patients (see chapter 11 for a case example concerning provider wellness). If you are a PCP, imagine that you are at the end of your career and your colleagues are giving you a retirement party. Your family members have come too, and now is the time when people are beginning to talk, one by one, about you and how you pursued your career, your work with patients and relationships with colleagues, and how you balanced your personal and professional lives. What do you hope they will say? (See appendix J, "Provider Tool: Retirement Party Worksheet.")

For patients, say this: "I want to better understand your values—what matters most to you in life—and a good way of getting at this is for you to imagine that you are at the end of your life and being laid to rest. What do you hope your loved ones will put on your tombstone? What would they say about you and how you lived your life?"

Bull's-Eye: Value Identification. If you like, you can use the Patient Education: Bull's-Eye Worksheet (appendix I and online) to introduce this exercise to the patient (see chapter 5 for a case example concerning chronic disease self-management). Explain that values are global, abstract concepts about what matters most to us in life, stating, "Values are like the bull's-eye on a dartboard; we don't usually hit the bull's-eye in a game of darts, but it gives us a direction. I'd like to know what your bull's-eye, or value, is in one of three areas today; you choose. Would you like to talk with me about your values concerning loving relationships, working, or playing?" When the patient responds, note the area of values focus on the handout, and then either write key words the patient says about her values, or have the patient write out the values statement. Often, you can end the visit by asking the patient to pay attention to times when she seems to be coming closer to the bull's-eye, just as a matter of what she does on a daily basis, and to come prepared to talk briefly about that at the follow-up visit.

Bull's-Eye: Value–Behavior Discrepancy. This exercise builds on the previous one and might be used during the same visit if time allows (see chapter 5 for a case example concerning chronic disease self-management).

Ask the patient to make a mark somewhere on the target on the Bull's-Eye Worksheet, to indicate how consistent her behavior has been with her stated value over the past few weeks. Total consistency would be the bull's-eye. It's important to explain to the patient, "Most of us are not hitting the bull's-eye but, rather, coming in somewhere out here" (pointing to one of the most distant rings). Sometimes patients respond, "Not even on the page." When this happens, let the patient know that it's okay and that the point of the bull's-eye is to create a focus so we can be more intentional in our day-to-day choices.

Sustain Value-Consistent Action

You are in an ideal position to help patients learn the skills necessary to make sustained efforts to live more mindfully and meaningfully. Sustaining value-consistent action relies on patients' ability to acknowledge that they can respond differently to troubling TEAMS and troubling external problems of living. It also requires that patients develop a better understanding of what choice means. Often, patients see their PCP as the ideal "witness" to their commitment to behavior change. The bull's-eye exercise in the previous section is a great metaphor to use to support patients in ongoing efforts to make behavior changes. We recommend using it with all of your patients to create real behavior change. You can print a copy of the Bull's-Eye Worksheet from the website (see also appendix I) and use one or more of the components of the technique (value identification and value–behavior discrepancy, discussed in the previous exercise) or the Bull's-Eye: Action Steps (described in the following exercise) at initial and follow-up visits with patients. We demonstrate use of the bull's-eye in most chapters.

TECHNIQUES TO SUPPORT ABILITY TO SUSTAIN VALUE-CONSISTENT ACTION

You Are Not Responsible; You Are Response Able. This exercise helps the patient sort out blame and fault, because they impact commitment to a course of action (see chapter 9 for a case example concerning trauma). Write the word "responsible" and then "response able." Explain to the patient that today we often associate "being responsible" with blame and fault. However, the original meaning of "responsible" was "being alive." Let the patient know that pursuing a life consistent with your values requires you to see the available options for responding in a vital, life-supporting way at any given moment in time and to choose that course: response able.

All Hands on Deck. This technique involves a metaphor (see chapter 7 for a case example illustrating use in a class for patients with chronic pain). When stressed, the mind calls out for help from all possible "hands," or resources. Unfortunately, the hands (our TEAMS) who show up may not be helpful after all, but instead hinder our ability to keep the ship on course. We think all hands should help us deal with challenges at sea (or difficulties we face in pursuing our values), but often some hands help and some don't; that is, some TEAMS help and others don't. The All Hands on Deck game helps the patient learn to continue pursuing a valued direction even when that pursuit causes more distress.

Invite the patient to be the captain of a ship, steering it toward a value direction, knowing that many negative TEAMS will emerge once the journey is under way. Have the patient name the TEAMS and command them, as "crew members," to come to the top deck to be ready to help out: "All hands on deck!" You can do this exercise in brief individual visits, but it works especially well during group visits, where group members can enact the metaphor. The targeted skill is to stay at the helm and continue steering, and this exercise allows the patient to experiment with how it works to argue with unruly or unskilled crew members, even making them walk the plank, versus acknowledging their presence while staying at the helm and steering the ship in its original direction.

Bull's-Eye: Action Steps. You can use the Bull's-Eye Worksheet (online and appendix I) or simply draw a bull's-eye on a piece of paper (see chapter 5 for a case example concerning chronic disease self-management). After the patient describes a value, ask him to identify one or more behaviors he could do that might bring his behavior on a daily or weekly basis closer to the bull's-eye value. Note steps—both short- and long-term—on the worksheet and give it to the patient to take home, requesting, "Will you, if possible, make a note or two when you try to do these things: how it went; what, if anything, got in the way? Then, you can bring it back, and we'll look at what the next step needs to be." If you decide to add a step or two concerning action steps for the patient to consider over the long term, note these and explain, "These are possible steps for us to ponder for the future." At a follow-up visit, ask the patient how the behavior-change plan worked. Did he do it? Did this process take the patient closer to the experience of vitality and purpose, as anticipated? What barriers did the patient experience? You and the patient can then revise the action plan, as indicated by the patient's experience.

 Burnout Prevention and Recovery Plan. This exercise is for students, residents, and providers of primary care services (see chapter 11 for a case example concerning provider wellness). Using this written exercise can help reduce the risk of burnout (see appendix L). When you complete this form, try to describe specific behaviors and details about when and how often you will use techniques to increase your resiliency. Planning areas on the worksheet include practice of acceptance, mindfulness, contact with personal values, and value-consistent action on a daily basis.

Use Observer Self to See Limiting Self-Stories

This process is about helping patients discover their "observer" self, the silent and consistent aspect of awareness that's present throughout life. It builds on the patient's ability to experience the self in the present moment, using the five senses. The observer perspective on self empowers the patient to better accept or "watch" sticky TEAMS without becoming embroiled in them and to persevere in valued action, rather than become lost in the past or future. It is the place where patients can learn best from direct experience and be freed, even if temporarily, from the rules that lead to ineffective action. This aspect of self is also the antidote for limiting the self-stories the reason-giving mode of mind generates. The "reactive mind" reacts to events, situations, and interactions by organizing them into cause-and-effect relationships and, on a larger scale, into self-stories.

TECHNIQUES TO ENHANCE ABILITY TO USE OBSERVER SELF TO SEE LIMITING SELF-STORIES

What Are Your Self-Stories? Ask the patient to try an experiment in order to get to know a different part of the self, a part we all have but are often unaware of (see chapter 9 for a case example concerning trauma). Then, ask the patient to write three to four sentences in response to each of the following situations:

- Imagine meeting someone you want to befriend and telling that person about yourself: "I am..."

- Imagine being falsely accused of something and needing to clear yourself: "I am..."

- Imagine applying for a job and telling the interviewer about yourself: "I am..."

When the patient returns, you can discuss differences among the self-stories and ask what part of the patient is the same in all stories. The answer is the part that witnessed the writing or telling of the story. Label that part as the "observer self."

Be a Witness. The concept of being a witness—for example, to a crime—is easy for patients to understand, and most can readily describe the qualities of witnessing as "watching, observing details, and so on" (see chapters 6 and 9 for case examples concerning alcohol and substance abuse and trauma). You ask the patient to be present (perhaps having taught the patient one of the techniques suggested for developing the first of the six core processes: experience the present moment) and to just witness or watch her uncomfortable thoughts, feelings, and memories. After the patient starts to witness or watch, suggest that she look at a troubling problem or decision and continue to witness. You might say, "Try using the words 'I am a witness for my thoughts, and I am having the thought that...'" Patients will also benefit from encouragement: "Noticing sticky thoughts and feelings in this way helps you stay present, so stay with it and also notice that you are the person right here and right now, the witness, who is aware of those thoughts, feelings, memories—whatever your mind offers up."

Circles of Self. This exercise helps the patient connect current distressing TEAMS with the witnessing self or "observer self" (see chapter 8 for a case example concerning anxiety and depression). To start this exercise, draw three circles. In the first circle, write a self-story and explain that this is the content, or TEAMS, that is pertinent to the patient's problem at the moment. In the second circle, write out the five senses and explain that these help the patient come into the present-moment experience of the self. In the third circle, write "observer self," and ask the patient to hold the piece of paper and to be an accepting observer who simply watches the story and the sensory experience. Sit in silence with the patient for two to three minutes and explain that practicing this exercise may help the patient learn to move among the circles of self more easily.

Miracle Question. This technique is quite useful in helping patients defuse and access a more open perspective (see chapter 8 for a case example concerning anxiety and depression). You may phrase the miracle question in a variety of ways; for example, "Let's pretend that while you are sleeping tonight, a miracle happens. You don't know what has happened, but on awakening in the morning, various things in your life have changed. You notice them as you go through the day. What do you notice first? What's different?" Or, you can be briefer: "Let's pretend for a moment that I can wave a magic wand and you suddenly feel better. What's different about you? What do I see that tells me you are feeling better?" If the patient responds negatively (for example, "I'm not losing my temper so much"), encourage him to reframe the response in a positive way (such as, "What are you doing instead of losing your temper?"). You need to encourage the patient to elaborate on his image of a better future. When a patient can access a more open perspective, he is more prepared to step back from limiting self-stories and take action one baby step at a time.

Step Back from TEAMS and Unworkable Rules

Fundamental to the other core processes, this process, (called *defusion*, in ACT terminology) involves developing the ability to look *at* thoughts rather than *from* thoughts, to recognize that thoughts are thoughts rather than *truths*. Just because we think something doesn't mean it's true. We call this "holding thoughts" rather than "buying thoughts." Our thoughts are words or pictures that help us solve many problems but create and maintain other problems. From a contextual behavior-change perspective, whether a thought is true or false is not important. Instead, we ask if a thought is useful in the sense of moving us in a valued direction. If not, we need to find a way to change our relationship with it, so that it does not interfere with our chosen course. There are numerous quick techniques PCPs can use to help patients learn about this process.

TECHNIQUES TO ENHANCE ABILITY TO STEP BACK FROM TEAMS AND UNWORKABLE RULES

Playing with Sticky TEAMS. In this technique, you invite the patient to develop a playful stance in response to thoughts or other TEAMS that tend to distress the patient and provoke avoidance and other unhealthy responses (see chapter 5 for a case example concerning chronic disease self-management). Here's an example: Have a patient who often buys a distressing thought put some music to the phrase (a favorite tune perhaps) and work up a dance, so that she can sing and dance the phrase, changing its control over her. Over time, the patient can learn to hum the tune when the thought or other TEAMS elements show up.

TEAMS Sheet. In this technique, briefly explain each of the TEAMS elements and then ask the patient to use the TEAMS Sheet to identify negative TEAMS that tend to "push" the patient around (see chapter 7 for a case example concerning chronic pain). Ideally, you will ask the patient to use it during the same visit in which it is introduced and then to practice sitting with the sheet at home for a few minutes every day. At the end of the brief home practice periods, the patient can jot down a few notes about the TEAMS he observed, bringing the results to you on a follow-up visit. Once the patient learns to use the TEAMS Sheet, you and the patient can use the sheet during visits, particularly when interaction between you and the patient may be under the influence of negative TEAMS that limit present-moment experience during the visit.

Velcro. This technique helps patients create some space around their most sticky TEAMS (see chapter 11 for a case example concerning provider wellness). Explain to the patient that we have many thoughts, feelings, memories, and so on, but that some appear to be "terribly important and worthy of immediate attention." These thoughts or feelings appear to have Velcro on them, so that they attach immediately to invisible Velcro strips on our foreheads. Once they are attached, we can no longer see them as just thoughts or feelings. If time permits, you can jot down a few of the patient's Velcro thoughts or feelings on sheets from a pad of sticky notes and hand them to the patient to place on her head or chest. The patient can take these with her and practice putting the Velcro thoughts and feelings on her head while standing before a mirror, and then taking them off and just holding them.

Clouds in the Sky. This exercise involves identifying troubling TEAMS and just noticing them when they show up, without evaluating them or struggling to change them in any way (see chapter 11 for a case example concerning provider wellness). As a way of cultivating this type of acceptance, you imagine lying under a shade tree and watching clouds in the sky. The goal is to place each TEAMS element on clouds drifting by, allowing them to reform and change, simply watching the ever-changing pattern.

Accept TEAMS and Focus on Action

This process builds on defusion, or being able to step back from TEAMS and unworkable rules, and it paves the way for committed action. It is the antidote for TEAMS avoidance. Acceptance entails making open and undefended psychological contact with our most unwanted TEAMS. Acceptance is not the same as resignation, hopelessness, or defeat. Instead, it is a choice to stand in the presence of distressing TEAMS, without attempting to control, suppress, or eliminate them. A closely related ACT concept is *willingness*, which is best thought of as a voluntary act of exposing yourself to a situation that is likely to trigger distressing TEAMS. Thus, often the first step of acceptance is being willing to enter a difficult situation rather than avoid it. The second step of acceptance is what you do when you get in that situation and distressing TEAMS arise. Willingness is often the first stem of a question you need to learn to use with your patients: "Would you be willing to _____ [enter some difficult TEAMS-producing situation—for example, "talk with your boss about a raise"], accept _____ [whatever difficult TEAMS you are working on with the patient—for example, feeling as if *There's no point in asking*], and behave in a way that's true to your values [for example, accept the thought, *There's no point in asking*, and ask anyway because it is consistent with valuing the quality of the services you provide]?" Our patients can truly begin to establish new life directions when they are able to defuse, identify values, plan actions, and experience and accept sticky TEAMS completely.

TECHNIQUES TO ENHANCE ABILITY TO ACCEPT TEAMS AND FOCUS ON ACTION

Eagle Perspective. Use the metaphor of an eagle, soaring high, to talk to the patient about the perspective that empowers us to plan a course and stick with it (see chapter 7 for a case example concerning chronic pain). An eagle headed for a nest notices a rabbit here and there, feels the shift in the wind, hears the screech of a red-tailed hawk, and continues to fly toward the nest. You might suggest that the patient simply take a deep breath and float up, letting go of both internal and external phenomena that distract from continuing on the chosen course.

Book Chapter. This technique helps patients begin to see their life narratives from an acceptance context, making it possible for them to have painful life experiences without letting such experiences "define" who they are (see chapter 5 for a case example concerning self-management of chronic disease). These experiences are part of a book in which no one chapter is more important than the other chapters. You could disclose, "I have lots of chapters in my life storybook; some I like and some I don't," while offering encouragement: "Maybe the chapter you are reading right now is called 'My Pain and Disappointments.' There are other chapters in your life storybook, maybe 'My Vision for Life,' 'My Best Moments,' 'People I've Loved,' 'My Spiritual Self,' and so on. Your life story isn't about one single chapter; it's the whole book. When the chapter about pain and disappointment comes up, try saying something like, 'Oh, this is the "Pain and Disappointments" chapter. I've read you before.'" You need to explain that it's important for us to honor every chapter in our life storybooks and to keep the "book" perspective.

Rule of Mental Events. This technique helps patients experience the paradoxical trap inherent in suppressing or avoiding painful TEAMS (see chapter 6 for a case example concerning alcohol and substance abuse). The rule of mental events refers to the fact that it's impossible to get rid of mental events and that, in fact, our attempts to suppress inside-the-skin phenomena actually result in the avoided event being more present. To help patients experience this, ask the patient to imagine an apple for a minute and then to make that image go away completely. Most patients will observe and see that, at best, they can change the apple from red to green (or some variation). Then, you can introduce the idea that the patient's efforts to control painful TEAMS are actually not working in the sense of making them go away and are, perhaps, only making the painful thoughts and feelings worse.

Lose Control of Your Feelings, Gain Control of Your Life. When using this technique, you may want to use the online patient education form associated with it. Alternatively, you can add a few features to the Bull's-Eye Worksheet (see chapter 6 for ideas on how to adjust the Bull's-Eye Worksheet for this technique and for a case example concerning alcohol and substance abuse). Basically, you will draw a box to the left of the bull's-eye and write inside of it, "Control your feelings? How? _____ " In a few words, describe what the patient does to avoid painful TEAMS (for example, drink alcohol or use drugs, or avoid going to certain places). Maintain a nonjudgmental attitude, perhaps saying, "I can see how you've settled on this. The problem is that you have only so much energy, and you can use it to control your feelings or to gain control of your life by choosing to live the way you want to. I am willing to help you gain control over your life. I will work with you, and we will plan small behavior changes that will help you live in a more meaningful way, making room for painful thoughts and feelings about _____." While saying this, you can draw a vertical line from the phrase, "Control your feelings?" toward the bull's-eye and write "Control your life" above and to the right of the bull's-eye, near the value statement box. Then, ask the patient, "What do you want to choose now: control your feelings or control your life? Then, you can enter into a discussion about the Value Identification component of the Bull's-Eye Worksheet.

SUMMARY

In this chapter, you learned basic behavior-change strategies you can start using today! Let's review the main points of this chapter:

- You can help patients shift from controlling what cannot be changed (such as painful TEAMS) to what *can* be changed (daily actions) by using the notion of workability.

- Workability refers to what the patient is doing to live a meaningful life and how it is working in the short and long terms. Some strategies work in the short term but then take us off-track in the long run.

- Psychological flexibility means being able to be present in the moment, fully aware and open to our experience, and to take action that's consistent with our values.

- Six core processes help create greater psychological flexibility, and, in this chapter, you learned a variety of techniques for helping your patients develop skills in each of these processes.

PREVIEW

Chapter 4 will introduce you to ACT-inspired tools that will help you accurately identify sources of psychological rigidity, quantify them, and develop quick and effective treatment plans using the Bull's-Eye Worksheet and the Real Behavior Change Pocket Guide (a list of the techniques described in this chapter and illustrated in the chapters in the second part of the book).

CHAPTER 4

Takin' It to the Streets: Real Behavior Change Tools

You can't see the future through a rearview mirror.

—Peter Lynch

To apply powerful principles of behavior change in your busy practice of medicine, you need a system that allows you to quickly and accurately discern your patient's struggle, identify the processes that contribute to inflexibility, and choose the interventions that would likely have an immediate positive impact. Although this may appear daunting at first blush, in reality, this new approach to behavior change is fairly simple and straightforward, and can—and has been—used in very brief primary care encounters. In this chapter, we offer tools for gathering information, assessing patient strengths and weaknesses (the Core Process Assessment Tool [CPAT]), and identifying techniques that target processes that support psychological flexibility (Real Behavior Change Pocket Guide). To augment the material in this chapter, we recommend printing the following four behavior-change tools (two interviewing tools and two treatment tools) from the website *before* reading further.

Remember, when this symbol appears next to discussions about a diagram or worksheet, you can find a copy online at http://www .newharbingeronline.com/real-behavior-change-in-primary-care.html.

Five Tools for Creating Real Behavior Change

Interviewing: Three-T (Time, Triggers, Trajectory) and Workability Questions, Love, Work, Play, and Health Questions

Planning and Providing Treatment: Core Process Assessment Tool (CPAT), Real Behavior Change Pocket Guide, Bull's-Eye Worksheet

INTERVIEWING FOR BEHAVIOR CHANGE

Creating behavior change in a time-effective manner begins with the ability to quickly assess the patient's life situation and to analyze which core processes are producing rigid responses and what an appropriate "target" of intervention will be. In what follows, we will provide you with some tips that will help you streamline the patient interview so that you can zero in on what's important rather than end up collecting a lot of useless information. Then, we offer two sets of questions to provide a structure as you learn to integrate these new ways of gathering information from patients.

Basic Interviewing Guidelines

The ultimate goal of a strong behavior-change interview is to compose an accurate description of the nature and course of the patient's presenting problem and to develop a "snapshot" of the patient's life space. To do this efficiently and repeatedly across patients requires following some basic interviewing principles.

SLOW DOWN

The pressure of fifteen-to-twenty-minute medical visits often tempts health care providers to jump on the first problem that's discussed and try to intervene immediately. This puts you in the position of intervening out of context. For example, if a patient with uncontrolled diabetes mentions difficulties with monitoring blood sugars, the provider may immediately try to help the patient develop a blood sugar monitoring plan. Unfortunately, what the patient may not mention is that the anxiety associated with seeing the "results" of the blood sugar reading is so intense that he avoids monitoring, to eliminate the anxiety. We encourage you to hold off and collect the necessary information to really know what's going on with the patient's TEAMS and the social context. If it takes more than one medical visit to collect this information, so be it. It's better to go slowly and be accurate than to rush to intervene with a lot of holes in your information array. Except in rare instances, the patient's "problem" is not going to go away between now and the next medical visit, so you can afford to be patient.

LISTEN WITH ACT EARS

Using ACT ears means listening for language clues that signal what the patient's change agenda is, what's being avoided, and what rules are being followed. If you develop this ability, you will quickly notice that most patients are not shy about giving you their version of what needs to change for things to improve. You might even ask, "What would tell you that your life situation has improved?" You will often hear things like, "I would have more confidence in myself," "I wouldn't be sad anymore," or "I wouldn't have these horrible memories." Basically, patients will tell you what they are avoiding if you go looking for it. Other language clues involve declaratory statements about difficult TEAMS (for example, "I just want to get rid of my anxiety," "I couldn't stand to talk to my spouse about our marriage because the pain would kill me"), loss of contact with life direction ("I just feel lost; I don't know what to do anymore"), or being in a losing battle with TEAMS ("I just can't get any peace of mind," "I'm so tired of struggling with this," "No matter what I do, I seem to feel bad"). Listening with ACT ears will allow you to quickly appreciate what the patient is avoiding and what the change agenda is, making it easy for you to redefine the patient's view of the problem in ACT terms.

A GOOD QUESTION IS WORTH A HUNDRED COMMANDS

To be a really good behaviorist, you need to be inquisitive, curious, interested, and nonlinear in your approach. This means that you ask a lot of questions and seldom direct the patient to do anything. Directive communications engender resistance, whereas questions signal interest and a wish to understand and help the patient. Telling an obese patient, "I recommend that you try to start exercising on a more regular basis to improve your health" will likely engender resistance. Asking the patient, "Would you be willing to experiment with exercising to see what effects it has on your health?" is a far softer and more patient-friendly way to get into the same discussion. Remember, when you are counseling your patient, try to find a way to take a recommendation or direct instruction you have in mind and turn it into a question that the patient can take hold of.

PRACTICE WHAT YOU PREACH

If you are going to teach your patients the skills they need to develop better psychological flexibility, you need to understand that you are role-modeling these skills during medical exams. Just as you are counseling a patient to accept troubling TEAMS, you need to show acceptance of the TEAMS that arise in you as well. If you want your patient to be in the present moment more often, you need to be in the present moment when you are with the patient. Believe it or not, patients do look at you as a role model, even in this crazy age of ultrabrief medical exams. If you show the same willingness to be open, aware, and engaged that you are asking of your patient, your impact on the patient will be more potent.

The Behavior-Change Interview Tool Kit

The real behavior change interview system consists of several parts, and we offer you tools to support your development of skills in all areas. The first involves completing a functional analysis of the problem concerning the patient. Functionally analyzing a problem means that you create a picture of antecedents (events, situations, or interactions that trigger the problem), responses (specific problematic behaviors), and consequences (positive and negative rewards following the behavior). To support your skill development for this part of the interview, we provide the Three-T and Workability Questions (appendix D). The second part of the interview involves going a little deeper into the behavior-change context by asking workability questions (motive, behavior, short- and long-term consequences). The goal for workability interviewing is to identify the patient's coping responses and sources of psychological rigidity that have surfaced. Remember that the impact of psychological rigidity is created in the behaviors (or lack thereof) the patient uses to address the presenting problem. The Three-T and Workability Questions provide the information you need to assess the patient's current functioning in core behavior-change processes that you will target in your behavior-change efforts.

For your new patients, we recommend also obtaining a "snapshot" of the patient's life context. Try using the Love, Work, Play, and Health Questions (appendix E) in your first visit with a patient, and depending on your available time, continue with the Three-T and Workability Questions or save them for a follow-up visit. In common parlance, think of the functional (the "Three-T" portion) and workability questions as the figure, and the life snapshot (the Love, Work, Play, and Health Questions) as the ground. Neither can be understood, functionally speaking, without reference to the other. Problem behaviors always are nested in a life context, and life contexts interact with, shape, and maintain problem behaviors.

THE THREE-T AND WORKABILITY QUESTIONS

The first goal of interviewing is to understand the presenting complaint, such that you have a very good feel for what triggered this problem, how long it has been going on, how it is evolving over time, what the patient has tried in terms of coping behaviors, and how coping behaviors have worked in the short run *and* the long run. Guidelines for types of questions to ask in this interview are presented in worksheet 4.1 (also appendix D). Think of the Three-T and Workability Questions as a tightly organized interview designed to give you a very clear picture of the problem (the figure) and to interest the patient in behavior change.

The Three-T Questions. These questions help create a reference point for your interactions with the patient throughout the exam. Believe it or not, one of the most common problems medical providers have is not getting a good handle on what the presenting problem really is. We will use the example of Ruby and Dr. Davis to illustrate how you can use the Three-T Questions to ferret out a masked presenting complaint, one where the patient is complaining of one symptom, but another problem is actually triggering the symptom (not uncommon in medical visits!). But, first, let's briefly review the importance of workability questions.

The Workability Questions. These questions help you determine what the patient has tried to solve or manage the presenting complaint, what degree of success the patient has achieved, and the unintended costs of these coping strategies. Most patients will have tried several things in an attempt to resolve the situation, so it's important to elicit as many of these strategies as the patient can recall. What you will see in these responses are the sources of psychological rigidity discussed in chapter 2. For example, you will want to assess how much trouble the patient is having with stepping back from TEAMS and unworkable rules. You will want to gauge the degree to which the patient is present and how identified the patient is with a losing self-story. Finally, you will want to get a feel for how connected the patient's coping strategies are with his values.

WORKSHEET 4.1
The Three-T and Workability Questions

Time	When did this start? How often does it happen? Does it happen at a particular time? What happens just before the problem? Immediately after the problem? How long does it last when it is present? Is it here all the time or is it episodic?
Trigger	What do you think is causing the problem? Is there anything that, or anyone who, seems to set it off?

Trajectory	What has this problem been like over time? Have there been times when it was less of a concern? More of a concern? Has it been getting better or worse over time? How about recently?
Workability Questions	What have you tried to cope with this problem? How have these strategies worked over time? Are you getting the kind of results you want? When you use this strategy, are you getting some accidental negative results in other areas?

In the following doctor–patient dialogue, Ruby comes to see her PCP, Dr. Davis, complaining of headaches that have steadily worsened over several months.

DR. DAVIS: When did your headaches start, Ruby? [Time Question]

RUBY: I've had headaches off and on over the years, but for some reason this has gotten real bad over the last several months—maybe six months or so.

DR. DAVIS: Did anything happen in your life about six months ago that might have set your headaches off? [Time Question]

RUBY: Well, the only thing I can think of is that my husband went back to vocational training school about—I think—seven months ago.

DR. DAVIS: Did this have an impact on you and your family? [Trigger Question]

RUBY: Yes, definitely. I have to cover more of the kids' activities and the household chores. I think the worst part for me, though, is that he's always preoccupied, and we have almost no time together anymore. I'm really not happy with my marriage, and I was before. I mean, it wasn't perfect but it was a good marriage.

DR. DAVIS: Okay, so this transition has changed a lot of things in your daily life; you have to cover the kids more, and you feel kind of out of touch with your husband. I have a few more questions about the headaches. When do they tend to happen? [Time Question]

RUBY: Usually in the evenings. I'm always tired, I haven't had time to relax, and then my husband just stays in the bedroom studying, ignoring the kids and me. I feel really annoyed.

DR. DAVIS: So, have your headaches been getting worse over the last several months? Are they happening more often, are they more painful, or do they last longer? [Trajectory Question]

RUBY: Definitely getting worse. I might have had one or two headaches a week when it started, even though they were really bad. Now, I have them pretty much daily, and I'm worried there might be something medically wrong with me. That's why I needed to see someone.

DR. DAVIS: Has there ever been a time in your life before when you had headaches, and if so, what tended to make them better or worse then? [Trajectory Question]

RUBY: As a matter of fact, I had headaches a lot during my senior year of high school. I was really stressed then. My parents were arguing a lot because our farm was failing, and I was trying to do well in school, apply for college—it was a difficult time. I'm not sure if anything made the headaches better; maybe getting out of the house helped. I would take long walks around the farm, and getting out in the fresh air seemed to help. I used to read to escape all of the stress, and that seemed to help. When I was at college, I didn't have any real trouble with headaches, even though I studied a lot and worked a part-time job.

In this very brief interview, Dr. Davis has established a close link among a household transition, related stress, and the appearance of Ruby's headaches. Talking about the headaches has opened the door to discussing a much deeper personal issue, namely Ruby's growing dissatisfaction with her marriage. Now, let's continue with the conversation between Ruby and Dr. Davis, as he transitions to the questions related to the workability analysis.

DR. DAVIS: Okay, so it seems that you are vulnerable to having more headaches when you are under a lot of stress, and now is one of those times. And one of the most stressful circumstances for you right now is not having any quality time with your husband. Am I on the right track?

RUBY: Yes, that's about it, and I really don't want to take medication for the headaches, other than over-the-counter ones when I really need them.

DR. DAVIS: Okay, so what have you done to try to improve your marriage while your husband attends school and works full-time? Have the two of you talked about this problem?

RUBY: No, I don't want to rock the boat. I promised to support his getting his degree. I just try to keep quiet and not feel so frustrated.

DR. DAVIS: How would you say it's working for you to stay quiet and avoid bringing this up with your husband? Do you think this is helping solve the problem?

RUBY: Well, when I think about it that way, I guess I'd say it's probably not helping my relationship with my husband, and I'm getting more frustrated and irritable with him.

DR. DAVIS: Okay, so rather than help solve the problem, it has the added effect of making you even more frustrated and irritable. What else have you tried to address the problem?

RUBY: Well, I don't want to feel angry and frustrated, because that isn't what I want to feel toward my husband, so I just leave the house and take a walk until I can get rid of this feeling.

DR. DAVIS: Does that work for you? Does it help you manage those negative feelings?

RUBY: It does for a while, but then he'll do something that feels thoughtless or inconsiderate, or he'll ignore something I say, and those feelings come back.

DR. DAVIS: So, would it be fair to say that leaving the house and taking a walk helps for a short time, but then the feelings return?

RUBY: Yeah. I also try to pretend I'm okay and that everything's fine when I'm around him, as if I'm not bothered. I learned

	to do that when I was a kid at home so my parents wouldn't have to deal with me.
Dr. Davis:	Has that helped solve the problem with your husband?
Ruby:	Even though I pretend I don't care, I do care, and it hurts when he doesn't pick up on the fact that I feel rejected by him. I guess that's my cross to bear in life: to be ignored and left behind by the people who are most important to me.
Dr. Davis:	It's clear to me that you really value your marriage, and you also value good communication and having a connection with your husband. You've tried a lot of things to address this problem with him, but none of them seems to be working very well; some of them, like leaving the house and pretending you don't care, actually seem to be making the problem worse. Is there anything you can think of that might have a better chance of working, of getting your marriage back on track?
Ruby:	I guess I should talk to him and tell him how I feel. I do need to have more time with him, not just time, I guess, but quality time, when we are both rested and interested in each other. My fear is that he won't care about my feelings, and he might even ignore me more if he gets angry with me.

This little vignette demonstrates that in a very short period of time (probably two to four minutes), Dr. Davis has extracted an amazing amount of information about what's working and not working in Ruby's situation, as well as identified many possible sources of psychological rigidity. Ruby's statements about not wanting to be angry and leaving the house to manage unwanted feelings suggests she is very fused with TEAMS and is following rules about them (for example, *You are not supposed to be angry at your spouse* and *Anger is a "bad" feeling*). Her main objective is to control her feelings of anger and frustration, which indicates that she has difficulty accepting negative TEAMS. Her strategy of pretending not to care and acting as if nothing is wrong is closely tied to her story of her childhood, and she has the same expectation of being unheard in her marriage. She is very identified with her self-story of going silent when she has needs that nobody she cares about notices. While her values for marriage seem to focus on intimacy and communication, her behaviors enact the opposite of those values. She is fused with a rule that says if she speaks out about her unhappiness, she is violating her obligation as a wife to support her husband while he is in school. Her basic coping strategies (silence and inaction) are passive and self-defeating. So, we have a number of negative processes contributing to her inability to effectively address her marital situation.

Using workability questions in a nonjudgmental, curious way tends to draw the patient out of "rule-following mode" and into "looking at the results" mode. Remember, workability is not about what *should* be working; it's about what *is* and *is not* working. Asking good questions about workability is a foundation for developing a good ACT intervention.

THE LOVE, WORK, PLAY, AND HEALTH QUESTIONS

This interview is divided into four sections: love, work, and play—but also health, because it affects these three important aspects of life. Love questions focus on the patient's living situation and the people who are a part of this context. Work questions concern study or employment (or alternative means of supporting oneself). Play questions concern the patient's recreational, relaxation, and social activities. We include questions about health-risk behaviors and health-promoting behaviors, as such can be liabilities or assets to the patient's functioning in the key areas of love, work, and play. See worksheet 4.2 for possible questions to ask during the love, work, play, and health interview (also see appendix E for an additional copy of the list).

Think of this interview as your attempt to create a "snapshot" of the patient's life in important life domains. The snapshot is the "ground" in the figure-ground relationship with the presenting problem, and given this relationship, you may sometimes ask the Love, Work, Play, and Health Questions *before* the Three-T and Workability Questions. The Love, Work, Play, and Health Questions are particularly useful when you are establishing a relationship with a new patient. When you ask these questions, most patients tend to relax and feel invited to disclose more personal information. This interview method is also helpful with psychologically distressed patients whom you might not know well, because these questions help you to better understand the context of the patient's decision to seek care, and they help you to learn about the patient's interests, abilities, and resources as a context for understanding the current problems.

WORKSHEET 4.2 The Love, Work, Play, and Health Questions

Love	Where do you live? With whom? How long have you been there? Are things okay at your home? Do you have loving relationships with your family or friends?
Work	Do you work? Study? If yes, what is your work? Study? Do you enjoy it? If no, are you looking for work? If no, how do you support yourself?
Play	What do you do for fun? For relaxation? For connecting with people in your neighborhood or community? Do you have friends? What do you do together?
Health	Do you use tobacco products, alcohol, or illegal drugs? Do you exercise on a regular basis for your health? Do you eat well? Sleep well?

Let's take the case example of Mr. Long to illustrate the use of this interview method in a brief visit with a new patient. Mr. Long is seeing his PCP, Dr. Jackson, with the complaint of a persistent cough over the last month. We will assume that Dr. Jackson has already completed a "Three-T" analysis of Mr. Long's cough.

DR. JACKSON [*while starting the physical exam*]: Where do you live, and who lives with you?

MR. LONG: I live about two miles from here. I moved here with my wife and two sons about a year ago—just haven't needed to see a doctor until now.

DR. JACKSON: Are things going okay at home?

MR. LONG: Well, yes, pretty good. We are tight for money, and the boys are teenagers, so I worry about them. But my wife and I, we both have jobs, so I'm thankful for that [coughs].

DR. JACKSON: What kind of work do you do?

MR. LONG: I work nights at the factory; I'm a shift manager. It's an okay job. I like the people I work with. Hope to get on the day shift soon.

DR. JACKSON: What do you do for fun and to relax?

MR. LONG: I do things with my wife and sons when I can. We have relatives here, and I go fishing with my brothers sometimes.

DR. JACKSON: Good. What about your health? Do you have concerns?

MR. LONG: Well, it's pretty good, but this cough hurts and keeps me from sleeping. I still smoke but want to quit. I did before, for a year, but started up again when I got the new job.

DR. JACKSON: If your values could speak, Mr. Long, what would they say about smoking?

MR. LONG: My values—well, to stop, and it's important for me to set a good example for my kids. My youngest is in junior high now, and he recently told me that one of his friends is smoking. The older one worries about me, and I would rather he look up to me.

DR. JACKSON: Mr. Long, can you talk a little more about being a good example, just what that means to you?

MR. LONG: You know, being healthy, being able to get out and throw the ball with the kids, laughing without going into a coughing fit.

DR. JACKSON: Sounds like being a good dad, a healthy, active dad, is one of the most important things in the world for you, Mr. Long. Have you exercised for your health on a regular basis during the past week or two?

MR. LONG: No, I just don't make time for it. Used to walk—now I just watch TV, putter around the garage. I'm working on an old car.

DR. JACKSON: Glad to hear that you exercised in the past. Do you get out in your community on a regular basis, maybe go to church or belong to a club?

MR. LONG: No, I used to help with the kids' baseball teams, but not in recent years.

As you can see, a PCP can use her own style in asking the Love, Work, Play, and Health Questions and jump-start a relationship with a new patient. An understanding of a patient's life context provides a positive foundation for discussing values and healthy behavior change. This information is critical to using the Bull's-Eye Worksheet, which we illustrate later in the chapter.

PLANNING AND PROVIDING TREATMENT

After you have used real behavior change tools to gather information, we recommend using the Core Process Assessment Tool (CPAT; appendix G) to get a picture of the patient's strengths and weaknesses in the six core processes of psychological flexibility and the pursuit of valued directions.

 ## The Core Process Assessment Tool (CPAT)

This simple tool helps you quickly assess a patient's functioning in each of the six ACT processes of rigidity and flexibility. Indicate your assessment for each process by marking an "X" on the line between the left side (greater rigidity) and right side (greater flexibility). If you like, you can use a rating scale, ranging from 0 (most rigid) to 10 (most flexible), which will allow you to calculate a total flexibility score (from 0 to 60). Using the CPAT on a regular basis provides you with a global impression of the patient's relative strengths and weaknesses and a sense of the person's progress over time.

Let's use Dr. Davis's ratings on the CPAT regarding his patient, Ruby (see sample worksheet 4.3). Concerning her ability to experience the present moment, Ruby tends to be a little overfocused on her past disappointments, and she's having some trouble staying present when negative TEAMS show up. At the same time, she can see a different way of approaching the situation in the here and now with her husband. Concerning her connection with her values, Ruby has lots of different values about marriage (wants to support her husband, to spend quality time together, to talk things through). On her ability to sustain value-consistent action, Ruby can express that there's a big discrepancy between her values for her marriage and what's happening in her marriage, and her behavior is inconsistent with her values. Rather than communicate with her husband, she pretends everything is okay when it isn't. In effect, there's a big disconnect between her values and her behavior. Regarding her ability to use the observer self to see her limiting self-stories, Ruby shows some ability to access her observer self to see her childhood story about her needs being ignored, but the story still drives her behavior in the present situation. As to her ability to step back from TEAMS and unworkable rules, Ruby is pretty stuck on negative TEAMS and unworkable rules that she shouldn't speak out and that anger is bad in a marriage. As to her ability to accept TEAMS and focus on action, Ruby appears to be actively avoiding TEAMS; most of her coping strategies are designed either to prevent being angry or to control and eliminate anger and frustration when it shows up. In sum, Ruby exhibits three clear sources of rigidity, any one of which an ACT intervention could target: she is fused with negative TEAMS and follows unworkable rules for dealing with them; she does not accept the presence of negative TEAMS, but instead actively tries to eliminate them by escaping the situation or by preventing them from occurring through pretending she is fine; and she acts in ways that are inconsistent with her values about living in a marriage.

SAMPLE WORKSHEET 4.3
Dr. Davis's CPAT Ratings Concerning Ruby

Six Core Processes: Psychological Rigidity	Patient Rating Today	Six Core Processes: Psychological Flexibility
Lives in the past or future	_____X_____	Experiences the present moment
Disconnected from values	_____X___	Has strong connection with values
Engages in impulsive, self-defeating action or inaction	__X_____	Sustains value-consistent action
Stuck in limiting self-stories	_____X_____	Uses observer self to see self-stories
Stuck in TEAMS and unworkable rules	__X_____	Steps back from TEAMS and unworkable rules
Actively avoids TEAMS	__X_____	Accepts TEAMS and focuses on action

The Real Behavior Change Pocket Guide

The Real Behavior Change Pocket Guide offers a list, by process, of the techniques described in chapter 3. We recommend printing a copy from the website (or copying appendix H) and laminating it, along with the CPAT. The Real Behavior Change Pocket Guide refers you to chapters where techniques are illustrated in case examples. If you focus on the patient problems that most concern you (for example, chronic pain or trauma), you will soon learn a variety of techniques useful with those patients. While you are learning, we recommend referring back to chapter 3 for a description of the various techniques you might want to try. You can implement each technique in as little as five minutes. Over time, you will learn most of the techniques and will no longer need to refer to the instructions in chapter 3 or the chapters that demonstrate use of the techniques in specific case examples. In fact, you will likely start to come up with some techniques of your own!

So, after making your assessment ratings on the CPAT, use the Real Behavior Change Pocket Guide in worksheet 4.4 to select a process to target and possible techniques to use to activate that process. In Ruby's case, she has already suggested something that's very consistent with her values about her marriage: to talk to her husband directly about her sense of disconnection and to actively try to schedule more quality time together. So, this would be "low-hanging fruit," as the old saying goes. She has already suggested it, so you might go in that direction with your intervention! Doing so will undoubtedly bring up her TEAMS fusion in the form of her branding emotions as "good" or "bad," so you might suggest that she simply describe her feelings without evaluating them. She will also have to be willing to have emotions like anger and frustration, and thoughts of being rejected, as she and her husband work through these issues over time. If she shuts down or disappears from the house when these feelings arise, she won't be able to live in accordance with her values in her marriage.

Ruby's case is a good example of picking an area of relative strength (strong connection with values) to help buttress other processes that are weak (TEAMS fusion, rule following, and TEAMS avoidance). In other situations, you might choose to directly target the weakest process, with the intent of building skillfulness in that area. For example, a patient with severe depression who appears numbed out might benefit from your directly asking what TEAMS the person is experiencing in that very moment, as a way to bring the patient to the present moment in direct contact with the emotions being avoided. The nice thing about using this approach is that you needn't worry about choosing the wrong process target, because work on one process nearly always stimulates growth in other areas.

WORKSHEET 4.4 The Real Behavior Change Pocket Guide and Instructions

Real Behavior Change Pocket Guide		
Six Core Processes: Psychological Flexibility	**Technique**	**Demonstration Chapter**
Experience the Present Moment		
	Time Line	8 (anxiety, depression)
	Three (or Five) Senses	8 (anxiety, depression)
	Balloon Breath	9 (trauma)
Strengthen Connection with Values		
	Retirement Party/ Tombstone	11 (provider wellness)
	Bull's-Eye: Value Identification	5 (chronic disease)
	Bull's-Eye: Value– Behavior Discrepancy	5 (chronic disease)
	Bull's-Eye: Professional and Personal Values Assessment	11 (provider wellness)
Sustain Value-Consistent Action		
	You Are Not Responsible; You Are Response Able	9 (trauma)
	All Hands on Deck	7 (chronic pain)

	Bull's-Eye: Action Steps	5 (chronic disease) 6 (substance abuse) 9 (trauma)
	Burnout Prevention and Recovery Plan	11 (provider wellness)
Use Observer Self to See Limiting Self-Stories		
	What Are Your Self-Stories?	9 (trauma)
	Be a Witness	6 (substance abuse) 9 (trauma)
	Circles of Self	8 (anxiety, depression)
	Miracle Question	8 (anxiety, depression)
Step Back from TEAMS and Unworkable Rules		
	Playing with Sticky TEAMS	5 (chronic disease)
	TEAMS Sheet	7 (chronic pain)
	Velcro	11 (provider wellness)
	Clouds in the Sky	11 (provider wellness)
Accept TEAMS and Focus on Action		
	Eagle Perspective	7 (chronic pain)
	Book Chapter	5 (chronic disease)
	Rule of Mental Events	6 (substance abuse)
	Lose Control of Your Feelings, Gain Control of Your Life	6 (substance abuse)

How to Use the Real Behavior Change Pocket Guide:

1. Print a copy of the pocket guide and keep it on a clipboard or in another place where you can find it easily at your clinic.

2. Refer to the brief descriptions of the techniques in this chapter as needed.

3. Study applications of the techniques in the case examples in the chapters indicated on the pocket guide.

4. Practice a technique (ideally with a colleague, a preceptor, or a friend) prior to using it.

5. When charting, indicate the process you targeted and the intervention you used.

6. With practice, you will become skillful at using a variety of techniques for each process.

Bull's-Eye Worksheet

The Bull's-Eye Worksheet is an ideal platform for supporting your patients in making real behavior change. We described three components of the bull's-eye behavior-change strategy in chapter 3 (value identification, value–behavior discrepancy, and action steps), and these, of course, are on the Real Behavior Change Pocket Guide. The Bull's-Eye Worksheet provides a structure for initiating and sustaining value-consistent plans for behavior change, and you can use any one or all three of the component techniques in any patient visit. As you work with it, you and your patient can identify barriers that arise when the patient attempts to implement behavior-change plans. Often, the barriers will link to one of the core processes of rigidity. You can then select techniques that may help the patient stimulate the corresponding core process of flexibility. In part 2 of this book, we use bull's-eye techniques with different types of patient complaints. As you read about bull's-eye applications to a variety of common problems in primary care, you will learn to apply this technique skillfully. Worksheet 4.5 provides a copy of the Bull's-Eye Worksheet, plus a guide to help you plan immediately prior to patient visits. You can print the Bull's-Eye Worksheet from the website, or copy appendix I. We recommend printing the worksheet and the Real Behavior Change Pocket Guide on double-sided paper and laminating them. With a dry-erase maker, you can use them repeatedly in patient visits.

WORKSHEET 4.5
The Bull's-Eye Worksheet

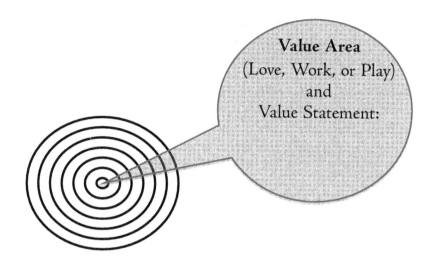

Value Area
(Love, Work, or Play)
and
Value Statement:

1	2	3	4	5	6	7
Not Consistent	Slightly Consistent	Somewhat Consistent	Consistent	Remarkably Consistent	Very Consistent	Bull's-Eye!

Action Step(s):

1.

2.

3.

Guide for Using the Bull's-Eye Worksheet

1. Ask the patient to choose love, work, or play as a focus for a short discussion about values. Have the patient explain what's important to him in each area of life.

2. Listen closely, reflect what you heard, and then write a statement on the Bull's-Eye Worksheet using the (global, abstract) words the patient used when talking about the value.

3. Explain to the patient that the bull's-eye on the target represents hitting your value target on a daily basis (and explain that most of us fall far short of that on a day-to-day basis, but knowing what the target is helps us make choices, set goals, and implement plans).

4. Ask the patient to mark an "X" on the target (or choose a number, with 0 being most distant from values and 7 being completely consistent with values) to indicate how close to the bull's-eye value statement her behavior has come over the past two weeks.

5. Ask the patient to plan one to three specific behavior experiments for the next two weeks that the patient believes will make his behavior more value consistent (closer to the bull's-eye target).

6. If time allows, rate the patient's current functioning level in one or more core areas on the CPAT (appendix G). This will provide a baseline against which you can judge the impact of the Bull's-Eye Worksheet.

7. If time allows, choose a core process area and a corresponding technique from the Real Behavior Change Pocket Guide (appendix H) to use in the visit.

8. At follow-up, ask the patient to re-rate value consistency (see step 4, above) and then to identify barriers to engaging in behaviors planned in the prior visit. Often, identifying barriers will point to the core process the patient needs to address in that visit to develop greater flexibility.

SUMMARY

In this chapter, we introduced the basic tools you need to create real behavior change over time. Let's review *and* plan for your development of mastery in using these tools:

- The interviewing tools are the Three-T (Time, Triggers, Trajectory) and Workability Questions; and the Love, Work, Play, and Health Questions (particularly useful in new patient visits). Print these from the website (or copy appendixes D and E) as a two-sided reference and laminate them.

- The tools for planning treatment are the Core Process Assessment Tool (CPAT) and the Real Behavior Change Pocket Guide. Print these forms from the website (or copy appendixes G and H) and laminate them.

- The Bull's-Eye Worksheet is the tool for providing ongoing care to patients who need your help to make and sustain behavior change. Print the Bull's-Eye Worksheet and the guide for using it from the website (or copy appendix I), as a two-sided reference and laminate them.

- Last, carry these three reference documents with you (as well as a dry-erase marker) at your clinic and use them often.

- One more thought: find a "buddy" who wants to improve patient outcomes *and* job satisfaction by using some of the latest behavioral interventions, and practice with that person.

PREVIEW

Chapter 5 begins the second part of this book. We will illustrate use of real behavior change tools in addressing chronic disease self-management.

PART 2

Promoting Real Behavior Change in Patient Care

This is where the rubber meets the road. In this part, we demonstrate how to use real behavior change tools to improve outcomes for problems that are often challenging in primary care: chronic disease management, alcohol and substance abuse, chronic pain, anxiety and depression, and trauma. As you may recall from this book's introduction, two bonus chapters are available online: "Angry Patients and Soft Eyes: Connecting with the Help-Rejecting Patient" and "You're Okay but Not for Long: Addressing Health-Risk Behaviors" (along with four additional patient education forms illustrated in the bonus chapters).

The Struggle: Engaging Patients with Chronic Disease

You can't get out of the room by moving the furniture.

—Source unknown

Though historically focused on treating acute problems, primary care providers now spend a great deal of time caring for patients with chronic conditions. Indeed, chronic conditions are the fastest growing part of primary care (Patterson, Peek, Heinrich, Bischoff, & Scherger, 2002) due to several factors, including an aging population; an increase in conditions like diabetes, lipid disorders, and obesity; and medical advances that allow people to live longer with diseases that would have been fatal in earlier years. The trend toward more chronic disease means that more patients must learn to cope with conditions that can disrupt lifestyles and relationships. While self-management practices—such as complying with a medication regimen and maintaining a healthy lifestyle—predict good outcomes, available estimates suggest that up to 60 percent of patients with chronic disorders adhere poorly to treatment (Dunbar-Jacob & Mortimer-Stephens, 2001).

Contextual behavior-change interventions can improve health outcomes with this large and growing group of patients. One of the most exciting findings in recent years involved a full-day ACT workshop for patients with diabetes. ACT strategies were integrated with standard educational materials about diabetes self-management. Compared with usual-care patients, ACT patients had better self-reported diabetes management and significant improvement in hemoglobin A1c measurement (Gregg, Callaghan, Hayes, & Glenn-Lawson, 2007). The *Diabetes Lifestyle Book* (Gregg, Callaghan, & Hayes, 2007) describes the ACT intervention provided in this study, and if you are interested in learning more about this innovative approach, we encourage you to buy the book and give it a try in your practice.

For now, let's consider the case of Ruth Ann and how Dr. Rosenthal, her family physician, uses behavior-change tools introduced in part 1. For each chapter in part 2, we identify specific process targets and demonstrate techniques that help the patient in the case example move toward greater psychological flexibility and more vitality. The box that introduces each chapter provides a summary of the tools demonstrated in the chapter. As you can see, in this chapter's introductory box, we reference the process on the Real Behavior Change Pocket Guide to help you refer back to chapter 3, where the six core processes of flexibility and techniques to activate them were introduced.

Chronic Disease Interventions

Love, Work, Play, and Health Questions

Three-T and Workability Questions

Core Process Assessment Tool (CPAT)

Real Behavior Change Pocket Guide

Process	Technique
Step Back from TEAMS and Unworkable Rules	Playing with Sticky TEAMS
Accept TEAMS and Focus on Action	Book Chapter

Strengthen Connection with Values	Bull's-Eye: Value Identification and Value–Behavior Discrepancy
Sustain Value-Consistent Action	Bull's-Eye: Action Steps

Remember, when this symbol appears next to discussions about a diagram or worksheet, you can find a copy online at http://www .newharbingeronline.com/real-behavior-change-in-primary-care.html.

CASE EXAMPLE: RUTH ANN AND DR. ROSENTHAL

Ruth Ann, fifty-three, had her most recent medical visit with Dr. Rosenthal's colleague nine months ago.

Reason for Visit. She presents for follow-up of diabetes mellitus II, hypertension, depression, and "feeling tired all the time." She was asked to come in to continue receiving refills on her medications and to see Dr. Rosenthal, who will assume responsibility for her care.

Medical Status. Other comorbidities include obstructive sleep apnea, gastroesophageal reflux disease, hypothyroidism, osteoarthritis (left knee, severe) and severe obesity. Her current nine medications include insulin and oral medications for diabetes. Her last visit was nine months ago, and her last HgbA1c was 9. She has gained some weight since her last visit.

Patient Concern. Ruth Ann is interested in getting her diabetes under better control and doesn't want to feel tired all the time. She hasn't been checking her glucoses regularly but knows they are high.

Patient's Life Context. Ruth Ann lives with her husband of eighteen years, who is also Dr. Rosenthal's patient. They have children and grandchildren who live in the area. She says she wants to be around for her grandchildren. She isn't exercising on a regular basis, does not eat breakfast, and rarely eats lunch. She drinks about three to four bottles of soda pop per day and relies on her husband to assist with completing household chores and managing finances. She ambulates within the household and does her own activities of daily living (ADLs). She doesn't smoke cigarettes, drink alcohol, or use any illicit drugs. She has difficulty getting up in the morning due to lack of motivation. She feels tired all the time and deals with this by going back to bed during the daytime.

Behavior-Change Interview

Dr. Rosenthal decides to use the Love, Work, Play, and Health Questions to enhance her understanding of Ruth Ann's life context and to introduce a discussion of values and the Bull's-Eye Worksheet. She also uses the Three-T and Workability Questions to focus the discussion on a meaningful behavior-change target. Sample worksheet 5.1 summarizes Ruth Ann's responses to the Love, Work, Play, and Health Questions.

SAMPLE WORKSHEET 5.1
Ruth Ann's Responses to the Love, Work, Play, and Health Questions

Area	Questions	Patient Responses
Love	Where do you live? With whom? How long have you been there? Are things going okay in your home? Do you have loving relationships with your family or friends?	Home of six years with husband of eighteen years Relationship okay; husband has health problems too, is sweet and brings me chocolate even though he shouldn't

Work	Do you work? Study? If yes, what is your work? Do you enjoy it? If no, are you looking for work? If no, how do you support yourself?	Unemployed for eight years Receive disability support, based on depression, diabetes, knee pain, and associated mobility problems Miss work—had friends there; have financial problems now
Play	What do you do for fun? For relaxation? For connecting with people in your neighborhood or community? Do you have friends? What do you do together?	Watch TV, do crosswords, listen to music Life centers around adult children, grandchildren in area Enjoy family gatherings on Sundays, cooking and eating
Health	Do you use tobacco, alcohol, or illegal drugs? Do you exercise on a regular basis for your health? Do you eat well? Sleep well?	No No No, no

This process helps Dr. Rosenthal in several ways. She understands for the first time that Ruth Ann lacks meaningful support for managing her diabetes. Her husband, her sole source of social support, is possibly contributing unwittingly to her difficulties with self-management. Dr. Rosenthal also has a better understanding of Ruth Ann's stresses related to finances and her loss of social opportunities when she became too disabled to work. Dr. Rosenthal also surmises that Ruth Ann's recreational and relaxation activities are sedentary and that her weekly social gatherings involve cooking and eating.

Dr. Rosenthal then shifts the conversation to the focus of the visit: Ruth Ann's interest in improving her skills for self-managing diabetes. Ruth Ann's responses to the Three-T and Workability Questions provide information necessary to form a doable behavior-change plan (see sample worksheet 5.2). Note that Dr. Rosenthal does not use all of the exact questions from the Three-T set, because she is adapting the list to her style and to her interaction with Ruth Ann.

SAMPLE WORKSHEET 5.2
Ruth Ann's Responses to the Three-T and Workability Questions

Area	Questions	Patient Responses
Time	When did you first start having trouble managing your diabetes?	Since diagnosis eighteen years ago
	How often are you aware of having problems managing your diabetes?	Daily
	Any recent worsening of symptoms?	Yes, difficulties with daily fatigue over past year
Triggers	Did something trigger its worsening?	"Just getting older, less active, fatter, too."
	What types of situations, events, or interactions make it more difficult to make healthy choices and follow through?	"Husband brings home bad snacks to get on my good side."
	Are there things inside of you that trigger this problem?	"I feel overwhelmed and just say to myself, 'forget it'!— Cat's out of the bag."
	How about things in the work or home setting?	"Husband says not to worry about my weight."
	How do you react when you notice that you are struggling to make healthy choices?	"I just eat a really small amount and try to have a good time, try not to think about it."
	How do others react to your problem?	"People stare at me."
	What do they tell you to do?	"They don't say anything, but I know they think I'm a pig."

Trajectory	Think about when you were diagnosed up till now; have there been times when you were better able to make healthy choices and stick with them? How about worse times? Is there anything you do that helps make the problem better now, even if temporarily? Anything that makes it worse? Do things that make it better in the short run make it worse in the long run (workability question)?	"Probably best when I still worked at the school—I was an educational assistant, and I liked it. I wasn't so fat then." "Seems like I get worse when I feel overwhelmed; I just give up." "I know that trying to ignore it and do what pleases me in the short run makes me sicker in the long run, and this makes me mad—well, more sad."
Workability Questions	What have you tried to cope with this problem? How have these strategies worked over time? Are you getting the kind of results you want? When you use this strategy, are you getting some accidental negative results in other areas?	"Distraction, I guess; just trying to think about something else." "No, not getting the results I want. I keep gaining weight and that makes me upset." "I guess what I'm doing just makes me more upset."

Dr. Rosenthal summarizes information from the Three-T and Workability Questions this way: "So, it's always been hard to manage your diabetes, and it's become more difficult since you left your job, with getting older and staying home most of the time. You did the best with it when you were working. What you're doing now—ignoring it—isn't working and actually makes you more upset, so you're ready to try something new." Dr. Rosenthal decides to introduce the Bull's-Eye Worksheet, hoping to initiate

93

a series of behavior-change visits. She hopes Ruth Ann will soon be willing to start attending her monthly Diabetes Lifestyle class for patients with diabetes.

Planning and Providing Treatment

To assure a good start to the behavior-change process, Dr. Rosenthal uses the CPAT to identify relative strengths and weaknesses. She decides to focus on two core processes: step back from TEAMS and unworkable rules, and sustain value-consistent action.

STEP BACK FROM TEAMS AND UNWORKABLE RULES

Dr. Rosenthal understands that Ruth Ann has several sticky TEAMS that she fuses with on a daily, if not hourly, basis, including the thoughts *Forget it* and *It's too late for me*, which come up when she feels tired or hungry. When Ruth Ann goes to the grocery, she struggles with feeling both deprived (*I can't have the things I want*) and guilty (*It's my fault I'm so big, and everybody knows it; they probably think I'm disgusting*). These TEAMS push her behavior around, leading to unhealthy behaviors such as overeating, eating the wrong foods, and avoiding going to the grocery.

Playing with Sticky TEAMS. This technique involves changing the context of a sticky thought. Basically, the idea is to say the word slowly or rapidly, softly or loudly, even to sing the troubling word or phrase—in other words, to play with it. Dr. Rosenthal explains this idea to Ruth Ann, suggesting that she experiment with responding more playfully to her *Forget it* and *It's too late for me* thoughts to see if this will help her to engage in behaviors that will improve her diabetes. Dr. Rosenthal explains that we sometimes take our thoughts too seriously and that we can free ourselves of them at times by simply shining a different light on them. She asks Ruth Ann to try singing "Forget it! It's too late for you!" to the tune of "Happy Birthday to You" to see if it changes the way she responds emotionally to these thoughts. Dr. Rosenthal warns that it will be hard to catch the thought at times, but that the more Ruth Ann tries to watch her thoughts, particularly in trigger situations, the better she will become at catching them and casting the "Happy Birthday to You" song spell on it.

Dr. Rosenthal also challenges Ruth Ann to play with sticky thoughts (such as *I'm fat*), perhaps saying them fast and then slow, in a whisper and then loudly. Dr. Rosenthal thinks Ruth Ann's learning to step back from sticky thoughts and unworkable rules (such as *Why bother? You always mess up anyway*) will empower her to initiate and maintain value-consistent action (for example, going outside for a walk or beginning the day with a healthy meal).

STRENGTHEN CONNECTION WITH VALUES

In an effort to help Ruth Ann more consistently pursue a meaningful life, Dr. Rosenthal decides to use the Value Identification component of the Bull's-Eye Worksheet.

Bull's-Eye: Value Identification. The Bull's-Eye Worksheet is useful for introducing this exercise. Share this form with your patient and explain that values are global, abstract concepts about what matters most to us in life: "Values are like the bull's-eye on a dartboard. We don't usually hit the bull's-eye in a game of darts, but it gives us direction. I'd like to know what your bull's-eye, or value, is in one of three areas today. Would you be willing to talk with me about your values? Let's focus on one area today. You can choose—maybe your values about love, work, or learning. Or you could choose to focus on your values about playing—having fun and feeling really alive. What seems most important today to you?" When the patient responds, note the area of value focus on the worksheet, and ask the patient to describe her value in that area. Then, either write key words the patient says about his values, or allow the patient to write out his own value statement.

Dr. Rosenthal asks Ruth Ann about her values concerning loving relationships with family members, because they are her central source of support. She asks Ruth Ann to "briefly describe how you hope your husband would see you as a wife, your children would see you as a parent, and your grandchildren would see you as a grandmother, if you were living according to your values." Ruth Ann explains that she wants her family members to see her as a "good person who is independent and able to take care of herself." She feels conflicted about having had to go on disability. She says she wants her family to also see her as a kind and generous person who goes out of her way to help others. On Sundays, when her large family comes to her house, she takes pride in always making an effort to help her grandchildren with school projects. As Ruth Ann responds, she seems more focused and alive, and Dr. Rosenthal records a few key words to describe Ruth Ann's values in her words. Then, as shown in sample worksheet 5.3, Dr. Rosenthal shares the Bull's-Eye Worksheet with Ruth Ann, reflecting, "This is it, your value, the bull's-eye for you—do I have it right?"

SAMPLE WORKSHEET 5.3
Ruth Ann's Bull's-Eye Worksheet

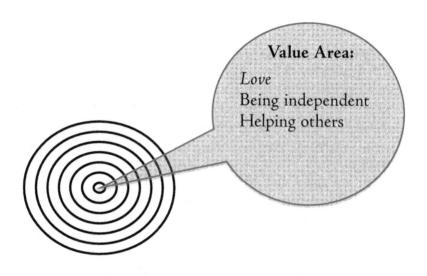

1	2	3	4	5	6	7
Not Consistent	Slightly Consistent	Somewhat Consistent	Consistent	Remarkably Consistent	Very Consistent	Bull's-Eye!

Bull's-Eye: Value–Behavior Discrepancy. This exercise builds on the Value Identification component, and it might be used during the same visit if time allows. Basically, you ask the patient to make a mark on the bull's-eye target to indicate how consistent her behavior has been with the stated value over the past few weeks. Total consistency would be the bull's-eye. It's important to explain, "Most of us are not hitting the bull's-eye but are coming in somewhere out here" (pointing to one of the most distant rings). Sometimes patients will respond, "Not even on the page," and when this happens, it's important to reassure the patient that that's okay and that the point of the bull's-eye is to create a focus so that we can be more intentional with our day-to-day choices. When Dr. Rosenthal uses this technique with Ruth Ann, the patient indicates she has not really been on the target, except for her decision to see Dr. Rosenthal and ask for help. Dr. Rosenthal suggests they use the rating box on the Bull's Eye Worksheet to track Ruth Ann's progress. Ruth Ann gives herself a baseline score of "1," for "Not Consistent."

ACCEPT TEAMS AND FOCUS ON ACTION

Dr. Rosenthal believes that Ruth Ann might be better able to sustain value-consistent action if she had skills that helped her accept difficult TEAMS while pursuing better self-management.

Book Chapter. This technique helps the patient begin to see self-stories from an acceptance context; specifically it helps the patient see that it's possible to have painful life experiences without having them define who you are in the present. Self-stories, the ones we like and the ones we do *not* like, are part of a book, and no one chapter is more important than another. Dr. Rosenthal introduces this idea to Ruth Ann and suggests that she has perhaps been spending a lot of time reading the "It's Too Late for You" chapter. Ruth Ann resonates with this idea, and Dr. Rosenthal wonders what other chapter titles Ruth Ann has in her book of life: perhaps the "Great Mom" chapter or the "Successful Tutor." In shifting toward bull's-eye planning, Dr. Rosenthal asks Ruth Ann to try naming book chapters she notices as she goes through her day to see how this helps her make healthier choices.

SUSTAIN VALUE-CONSISTENT ACTION

Dr. Rosenthal helps Ruth Ann move toward an action plan, beginning with a few small steps.

Bull's-Eye: Action Steps. You can use the Bull's-Eye Worksheet (appendix I) or simply draw a bull's-eye on a blank piece of paper. In using the Action Steps component of the Bull's Eye Worksheet, you ask the patient to identify one or more steps he could take that might bring his daily or weekly behavior closer to the bull's-eye value. Note these possible action steps on the worksheet and give it to the patient to take home, requesting, "Will you, if possible, try one or more of these steps and also note what happens when you try these things: how it went and what, if anything, got in the way? Then, bring it back, and we'll look at how these steps worked for you and perhaps identify other action steps." At a follow-up visit, ask the patient if he tried one or more of the action steps. If he did, what exactly did he do, and did it seem to bring him closer to his value? If it did, encourage him to continue with that action. If it didn't bring him closer to his value, help him identify other steps that are more likely to enhance value consistency. If he didn't take a step, what got in the way? The patient's answers will help you identify processes that pull the patient toward rigidity. As you work, make notes on the Bull's-Eye Worksheet so the patient has a reference. At times, you may indicate both short-term and long-term action steps on the worksheet. Often, you may elect to note only short-term action steps.

After talking briefly about action steps, Ruth Ann and Dr. Rosenthal plan several steps and note them on the Bull's-Eye Worksheet. Ruth Ann's action steps include both short- and long-term plans. See sample worksheet 5.4 for details. (To assist with your learning, we note the name of the most pertinent core processes of flexibility after each action step. This will help you begin to see the link between behavior change plans and ACT core processes that support behavior change.) While the first two action steps require Dr. Rosenthal to provide coaching during the visit, the third and fourth are added to the list without an extensive explanation. Dr. Rosenthal simply says, "Let's try two other things, just to see what happens." It is not necessary to explain that monitoring the behavior of breakfast eating requires some present-moment skills or that walking around the house will present Ruth Ann with the challenge of accepting difficult TEAMS (such as *It's too late for you*). At times, patients surprise their PCPs by demonstrating skills in processes activated by behavior change plans. At other times, they struggle. When the patient does not succeed, it's an opportunity for you and the patient to explore the barrier, identify the core process, and apply a new behavior-change technique. In ending the visit, Dr. Rosenthal makes a note on the Bull's-Eye Worksheet concerning the Diabetes Lifestyle class and explains that she will tell Ruth Ann about it at her next visit.

SAMPLE WORKSHEET 5.4
Dr. Rosenthal and Ruth Ann's Bull's-Eye Worksheet

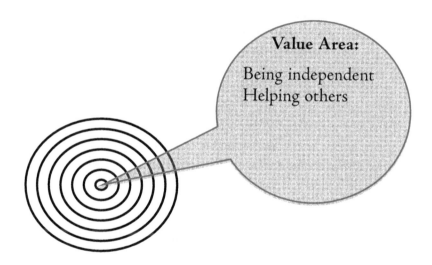

Value Area:

Being independent
Helping others

Action Step(s) (Short-Term):

1. *When you notice the thought "forget it," sing it to tune of "Happy Birthday to You" (Step Back from TEAMS and Unworkable Rules).*

2. *Look at your bull's-eye value statement every morning (Strengthen Connection with Values) and remind yourself to watch your life's "Book Chapters" that you notice throughout the day.*

3. *Monitor whether or not you eat breakfast (Experience the Present Moment).*

4. *Experiment: Can I think about being fat and still go out and walk around the house (Accept TEAMS and Focus on Action)?*

Action Step(s) (Long-Term):

1. *Possibly join monthly diabetes class (Sustain Value-Consistent Action).*

Providing Follow-Up Care to Ruth Ann

Ruth Ann comes for two follow-up visits and then joins Dr. Rosenthal's monthly Diabetes Lifestyle class. In the first follow-up visit, Ruth Ann reports having started a routine of going out for a walk around the house (and sometimes her yard) every morning and afternoon, and of singing "Forget it!" to the tune of "Happy Birthday to You" at the beginning of the walk. She eats oatmeal every morning for breakfast after her walk and is actually starting to enjoy it, because she has more of an appetite after her walk. During her walks, she finds herself thinking about how much better her life was when she was working. She decides she wants to find a way to help children and has invited one of her grandchildren to come after school on Wednesdays to work on his reading skills. She indicates that her husband voiced some concern about her walks ("What if you fell down or got to hurting badly and didn't have a place to sit?"), but she insisted that she is improving her physical condition and stamina by continuing to walk. Dr. Rosenthal acknowledges her independence and follow-through. She suggests that Ruth Ann bring her husband to a follow-up visit in two weeks, so that they can talk about their values as a couple and how health fits into those. Ruth Ann agrees to continue with the behavior changes she has initiated and to have several talks with her husband concerning their values about being playful and experiencing a variety of pleasures in life.

Ruth Ann and her husband, Sam, come to the next appointment and briefly talk about their values concerning play and pleasure. In the past, the two enjoyed going to the river and to the mountains to look at plants and do some bird-watching. They both agree that it would be nice to restart these activities. Sam is no longer concerned about Ruth Ann's walks and is, in fact, joining her for a walk around the block occasionally. During the visit, Dr. Rosenthal asks the two to brainstorm ways to show each other caring and love on a daily basis. When Sam says he likes to bring Ruth Ann a doughnut when he goes to the grocery, Ruth Ann responds she would prefer that he say, "I love you," or ask her to sit on the porch with him instead. Ruth Ann agrees to begin attending the monthly Diabetes Lifestyle class and to continue with the behavior changes she has initiated.

In her first class, Ruth Ann talks easily with others in the group, sharing her recent success in improving her lifestyle and listening attentively when others speak. She also appears to be interested in learning about the research on medication Dr. Rosenthal discusses toward the end of the class. At the conclusion of the class, Ruth Ann voices a plan of working toward regular testing of her blood sugars. One of the other patients indicates she is working on this as well, and she gives Ruth Ann her phone number, suggesting they could be testing "buddies."

SUMMARY

Congratulations! You have completed the first chapter of applying ACT to high-impact primary care patients.

- You've learned to use all components of the Bull's-Eye Worksheet (Value Identification, Value–Behavior Discrepancy, and Action Steps) to help your patients with chronic disease. Remember that the Bull's-Eye Worksheet is a useful support for these techniques (see appendix I).

- You also learned how to apply the Playing with Sticky TEAMS technique.

- Remember that you can use real behavior change techniques in groups for patients with diabetes (and *The Diabetes Lifestyle Book* [Gregg, Callaghan, & Hayes, 2007] offers you an evidence-based curriculum).

PREVIEW

In the next chapter, you will learn to apply behavior-change techniques to patients who are struggling with alcohol and substance abuse problems.

CHAPTER 6

The Solution That Becomes the Problem: Intervening with Alcohol and Substance Abuse

Here's to alcohol: The cause of, and solution to, all of life's problems.

—Homer Simpson

Alcohol and drug abuse and dependence are common problems that have numerous adverse effects on the health of our patients and their loved ones. Men are four times more likely to be heavy drinkers, and Hispanics are most likely to engage in heavy alcohol use, followed by Caucasians and African Americans (Schneider Institutes for Health Policy, 2001). More than 75 percent of domestic violence victims report that their assailants had been drinking or using illicit drugs at the time of the incident, and children from families with substance-abusing parents are more likely to have problems with delinquency, poor school performance, and emotional difficulties than their peers from homes without substance abuse (ibid.). Excessive alcohol use is responsible for a hundred thousand deaths annually, and alcohol abuse costs nearly $166 billion each year (ibid.). PCPs work diligently to detect problems with alcohol and drug abuse and intervene.

From an ACT perspective, alcohol and a variety of prescription and street drugs offer patients the option of immediate and (often) complete avoidance of painful TEAMS (most commonly from such things as traumatic memories; chronic negative emotional states; physical pain; ruminative, racing thoughts; or some combination of these). The effect of alcohol or drugs is to numb acute psychological pain. This pattern of escape and avoidance often widens over time and begins to grab hold of the patient's life space. Problematic use of alcohol and drugs creates additional life stresses (including powerful urges to use) that in turn produce more negative TEAMS, which require more numbing behavior. The downward spiral into addiction is complete when the patient is living a life organized around using drugs or alcohol, rather than a life based on personal values and valued actions.

However, there's reason to hope that ACT can help us improve our outcomes with patients who are sliding into avoidance patterns involving problematic use of drugs and alcohol. In a recent study, patients receiving ACT interventions, compared with a standard 12-step program, had better outcomes at the twelve-month follow-up (Hayes, Wilson, et al., 2004). Specifically, patients receiving ACT treatment demonstrated a decrease in the number of days they used drugs and in the amount of drugs used.

Let's consider the case of Luis and see how Dr. Young, his family physician, applies ACT. The following table summarizes ACT methods demonstrated in this chapter. We target three processes and demonstrate four techniques in this case example, as you can see in the chapter introduction box.

Substance Abuse Interventions

Love, Work, Play, and Health Questions

Three-T and Workability Questions

Core Process Assessment Tool (CPAT)

Real Behavior Change Pocket Guide

Process	Technique
Accept TEAMS and Focus on Action	■ <u>Lose Control of Your Feelings, Gain Control of Your Life</u> ■ The Rule of Mental Events
Use Observer Self to See Limiting Self-Stories	Be a Witness
Connect with Values and Sustain Value-Consistent Action	<u>Bull's-Eye Worksheet</u>

Remember, when this symbol appears next to discussions about a diagram or worksheet, you can find a copy online at <u>http://www .newharbingeronline.com/real-behavior-change-in-primary-care.html</u>.

CASE EXAMPLE: LUIS AND DR. YOUNG

Luis, a thirty-six-year-old Mexican American male, is an established patient of Dr. Young who visits the doctor so rarely that he hasn't been seen in the past twenty months.

Reason for Visit. His coworkers brought him to the clinic today because he "almost passed out at work this morning and looked very pale." He complains of dizziness. The weather has been very hot lately, with temperatures around 100 degrees Fahrenheit.

Medical Status. Luis reports good health and explains that he brings a quart of water with him to work but does not eat anything before he starts his workday. He is overweight but free of diagnosed chronic diseases, and he doesn't take any prescribed or over-the-counter medications. His physical exam is within normal limits (WNL). His complete blood count (CBC) is normal, but his chemistry panel shows elevated liver function tests. His family history is positive for alcoholism in his father.

Patient Concerns. Luis is worried about passing out or losing his balance while doing orchard work, because this could be dangerous. He also complains of insomnia, mainly difficulties with waking up too early and being unable to get back to sleep. He complains that he often doesn't "feel right" in the morning.

Patient's Life Context. Luis works as a farm laborer, is married, and has four children. His wife does not work outside the home. He has three brothers and three sisters who live in the area. Most of his social activities are with his family or coworkers. He doesn't exercise, stating that his work is his exercise. He doesn't smoke but drinks an estimated four to six beers a day and sometimes mixes in hard liquor on days off. He is not sure how much he drinks on weekends but says it's more than when he is working. Much of his drinking is with coworkers after work or with his brothers on weekends. He likes to spend his leisure time having a few beers; occasionally, he plays with his children, goes to movies, or goes grocery shopping with his wife. He and his wife disagree about whether his drinking is a problem. He thinks it's normal for his peer group; she thinks it's causing him to gain weight and be unhealthy. Luis left home at age sixteen to get away from his father; he describes his father as a heavy drinker who was critical of him and violent toward his mother. His mother died four years ago in an accident involving a drunk driver. His mother and father had divorced roughly six months earlier, when his mother discovered his father had been involved with another woman for several years during their marriage.

Behavior-Change Interview

Dr. Young is concerned that Luis might be developing a physical and emotional dependence on alcohol, so she wants to further clarify the impact his drinking is having on his ability to function at work and at home. Sample worksheet 6.1 summarizes Luis's responses to the Love, Work, Play, and Health Questions.

SAMPLE WORKSHEET 6.1
Luis's Responses to the Love, Work, Play, and Health Questions

Area	Questions	Patient Responses
Love	Where do you live? With whom? How long have you been there? Are things going okay in your home? Do you have loving relationships with your family or friends?	Married fifteen years; wife and four children at home. Same home for four years. "Wife nags me about drinking, causes arguments." "Stopped having sex a while back." Like being with kids sometimes, but often too tired or distracted.
Work	Do you work? Study? If yes, what is your work? Do you enjoy it? If no, are you looking for work? If no, how do you support yourself?	Like working in the fields and make good money. "I take pride in doing a good job, like being with my buddies and relaxing at the end of the day." Have not missed work because of drinking.

Play	What do you do for fun? For relaxation?	"Be with my family, sometimes go fishing or to the park with my family." "Watch TV, have a few beers."
	For connecting with people in your neighborhood or community? Do you have friends? What do you do together?	Stopped going to church after moving out of parents' house. "We drink, watch TV, sometimes go fishing." "My wife is always going somewhere with the kids."
Health	Do you use tobacco, alcohol, or illegal drugs?	"I drink, six or so beers after work; smoke on occasion, when someone else is smoking—I don't buy cigarettes or nothing like that."
	Do you exercise on a regular basis for your health?	"I work in the fields—hard —all day."
	Do you eat well? Sleep well?	"I eat okay, sometimes miss breakfast, but I don't sleep so well. I wake up a lot."

This brief interview helps Dr. Young understand that Luis's drinking is beginning to have a negative impact on his relationship with his wife and children and perhaps with his willingness to participate in activities outside the home that conflict with drinking. Dr. Young also realizes that Luis is likely to get little support or might even be ridiculed by his coworkers if he cuts back or stops his drinking.

Dr. Young is curious about how Luis got started drinking in the first place, what sorts of triggers elicit his drinking, the ebb and flow of his drinking problems over time, and what TEAMS he avoids or numbs through drinking. Luis's responses to the Three-T and Workability Questions help Dr. Young understand the context of Luis's drinking (see sample worksheet 6.2).

SAMPLE WORKSHEET 6.2
Luis's Responses to the Three-T and Workability Questions

Area	Questions	Patient Responses
Time	When did you first start to have trouble with drinking?	Four years ago. "My parents divorced, then my mother died in a car accident; the driver of the other car was drunk. I never drive when I drink—never."
	Are you drinking more now than you used to?	"I only had a few beers now and then before my parents divorced and Mom died; I guess I didn't want to be like my dad."

Triggers	Did something trigger its worsening?	"After Mom died, I think I was so angry at my Dad I wanted to kill him; I didn't want to feel that way; it didn't help anything."
	What types of situations tend to make you want to drink more?	"When my wife criticizes me or threatens to leave and, I guess, when I snap at the kids. I hate to do that."
	Are there things inside of you that trigger this problem?	"Lots; feels like a volcano sometimes; I hate it." Anger, grief, sadness, anxiety. Has trouble fighting urges to drink; attempts to ignore them don't work. Drinks during fights with wife.
	How about things at work that make you want to drink?	"My buddies and just feeling tired and achy, but all wound up, at the end of the day."
	How do you cope with the urge to drink?	"More and more, I think I just drink if it's available; I do try to limit myself to one six-pack a day sometimes."
	How do other people react to your drinking?	"I think people are getting worried about me, and I'm a little worried too; it really makes me feel bad, the way my kids look at me sometimes when I'm loaded."

Trajectory	During the past four years, have you done better with drinking sometimes and worse at others?	"Pretty much, just more and more over the past four years."
	Is there anything you do that helps make the problem better, even if temporarily?	"Play with kids or something, maybe eat before I have the first beer. Other than that, I guess I just try to hide it from the wife and kids, put my beer in a water bottle, you know, so they don't get cranked up."
	Anything that makes it worse?	"I drink more when I'm alone." Trying to ignore urges makes them stronger.
	Do things that make it better in the short run make it worse in the long run?	"I'd say that hiding it from the family and pulling back from them doesn't work, and look at me—my buddies brought me in 'cause I couldn't work; it's starting to affect my body."
Workability Questions	What have you tried to cope with this problem? How have these strategies worked over time? Are you getting the kind of results you want? When you use this strategy, are you getting some accidental negative results in other areas?	"I'm not handling my feelings or my drinking very well. And I am hurting my wife and kids with what I'm doing."

Dr. Young summarizes her findings in the following way, hoping to avoid stigmatizing Luis and, instead, emphasizing the many positive opportunities in this situation: "I'm so glad you came in to see me today, because you have the opportunity to do something very special for you and your family. You can develop new ways to deal with the death of your mother and your painful emotions about your father, your relationship with your wife, and other things that are bothering you. It seems that you have discovered that drinking helps you control these feelings, but at the cost of being unable to be the father you would like to be for your kids. Also, it seems that drinking has driven a wedge between you and your wife, and this bothers you so much that you have to use alcohol to control those feelings too. If, together, we can find another way to deal with these difficult emotions, I'm sure you will find a way to be the kind of person you want to be."

Planning and Providing Treatment

Dr. Young wants to help Luis directly experience the basic problem he is facing. If Luis is unable to accept his painful feelings for what they are (painful but normal human emotions), he will continue to avoid, suppress, or numb them through drinking. The cost of this avoidance strategy is that it takes him farther away from living the way he wants to. Drinking alcohol to avoid an experience is not a value-consistent behavior for Luis. Dr. Young decides to focus her intervention on three processes: ability to accept TEAMS, use observer self, and take value-consistent action.

ACCEPT TEAMS AND FOCUS ON ACTION

Dr. Young uses a technique designed to help patients see the lure of alcohol: alcohol offers a powerful, readily available, and reliable vehicle for avoidance. She chooses this technique because she believes it will help Luis begin making more intentional choices about drinking.

 Lose Control of Your Feelings, Gain Control of Your Life. Dr. Young shows Luis the Bull's-Eye Worksheet and writes a few key words in the Values Area. Then she summarizes the situation: "You are a person who very strongly believes in being a loving, caring father and husband. You are trying to aim your life so that you hit the center of the bull's-eye; that's your value, what matters to you. You get drawn off course by your painful thoughts and feelings about your dad and about your mom's death. You've found a way to control them—by using alcohol to numb out." Then, she draws a box to the left of the bull's-eye and writes, "Control your feelings: Use alcohol to numb out." She continues to explain his choice: "You have only so much energy, Luis. You can use it to control your feelings by numbing out, or you can use it to gain control of your life by choosing to live the way you want to. I am willing to help you gain control over your life. I will work with you, and we will plan small behavior changes that will help you live in a more meaningful way, making room for your painful thoughts and feelings about your parents." Sample worksheet 6.3 provides a picture of the way this acceptance-promoting technique is used with Luis.

SAMPLE WORKSHEET 6.3
Patient Education: Lose Control of Your Feelings, Gain Control of Your Life

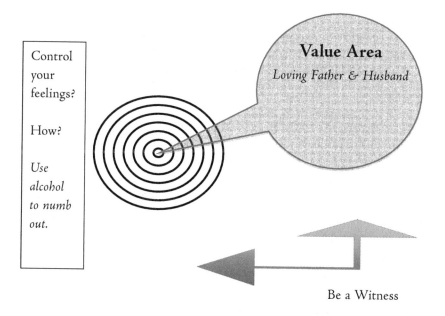

Control your feelings?

How?

Use alcohol to numb out.

Value Area
Loving Father & Husband

Be a Witness

Rule of Mental Events. Dr. Young also wants Luis to understand that he is caught in a paradoxical trap, and to achieve this goal, she explains the Rule of Mental Events to him. This rule refers to the fact that we cannot get rid of TEAMS and that attempts to suppress or avoid them actually result in their being more present. Dr. Young provides this brief explanation to him: "Luis, if you think about the painful feelings you've experienced over the years since your mother and father divorced, and your mother died, do you think your feelings have become less painful as a result of drinking to help control them, or do you feel that things have gotten worse?" Luis replies that his painful memories and emotions seem to be happening more often, even though he is drinking. Dr. Young responds, "So, you are not really controlling these feelings by drinking; they are actually getting worse? It sounds as if you are caught in a kind of trap where the harder you try to control the way you feel, the worse your feelings get."

USE OBSERVER SELF TO SEE LIMITING SELF-STORIES

Because Dr. Young is short of time, she uses the Be a Witness intervention rather than the Circles of Self exercise. She plans to link the experience of "witnessing" to help Luis make an intentional choice about whether to lose control of his feelings to gain control of his life, or the alternative (lose control of his life by controlling his feelings through problematic use of alcohol).

Be a Witness. Dr. Young wants to propose an alternative strategy to Luis, one that will require him to abandon his ongoing attempts to control his painful TEAMS. She wants to see whether he is willing to just observe his emotions without doing anything to control them. "I wonder what would happen if you tried a different strategy, to accept that you have these painful emotions and to just let them be there without needing to do anything to change them? Your emotions don't define who you are, any more than wearing a particular shirt or pair of pants does. It's the same with urges to drink: they get their power from your struggling to control them; doing so makes them bigger, not smaller. Maybe when you have these negative memories and feelings about your mother and father, or start to experience urges to drink, you could just witness them." At the bottom of sample worksheet 6.4, she writes, "Be a Witness."

Dr. Young realizes it is probably too early to talk to Luis about quitting drinking altogether, given his history and the social pressure in his peer group. Instead, she suggests discussing "mindful drinking" at his follow-up visit and explains that using more of the "witness" approach whenever he drinks might also help. She says that other patients report that this approach helps them slow down their drinking, allowing for more choice in the matter.

CONNECT WITH VALUES AND SUSTAIN VALUE-CONSISTENT ACTION

Given the chronic nature of Luis's problem, Dr. Young uses the Bull's-Eye Worksheet.

Bull's-Eye Worksheet. As described in the previous chapter, the Bull's-Eye Worksheet helps you collaborate with the patient in developing one or two action steps the patient can take to see if he can increase the connection between his stated values and daily behavior. Luis indicates that his drinking is not consistent with his values, and the visit ends with completion of the Bull's-Eye Worksheet (see sample worksheet 6.4). He agrees to return in two weeks.

SAMPLE WORKSHEET 6.4
Dr. Young and Luis's Bull's-Eye Worksheet

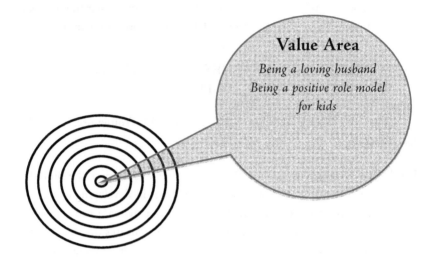

Value Area

Being a loving husband
Being a positive role model
for kids

Action Step(s):

1. *When you notice emotions about your mother, father, or family problems, consider the choice to just witness them (Use Observer Self to See Limiting Self-Stories).*

2. *When urges to drink arise, sit motionless for five minutes and just witness, or observe, them before getting a drink (Use Observer Self to See Limiting Self-Stories).*

3. *Try to schedule one positive activity with wife and children each weekend day at a time when you normally drink (Sustain Value-Consistent Action).*

Providing Follow-Up Care for Luis

Luis returns in two weeks, as planned, this time accompanied by his wife. They both agree that Luis is doing better. He is drinking less on weeknights and weekends. He has had no further problems with dizziness, feels better in the mornings, and is even sleeping a little better. On two consecutive weekends, the family has gone out for a fun activity. Luis says he really enjoyed himself and feels he is more consistently living his value of being a good role model for his kids. Luis finds it especially hard, however, to simply witness his anger toward his father. He agrees that he has carried this emotion around for a long time and it will take time to simply allow it to be there without letting it "push me around." He does succeed in just observing his sadness and grief over his mother's death, and he actually cries about her for the first time in several years. He struggles with drinking excessively when hanging out with his brothers at family parties, because they often drink too much, too. Dr. Young talks with Luis about mindful drinking, and they agree to the following addition to his action steps:

> **New Action Step:** *Mindful drinking, involving taking five minutes between sips of beer or hard stuff; savor the taste, texture, and temperature, noticing what's going on inside and outside your body as you do this (Experience the Present Moment).*

Luis returns alone in two weeks and looks visibly healthier. He is sleeping better, and he and his wife are being intimate again. Though he found the mindful-drinking exercise difficult, he plans to continue with it. He has signed up to be an assistant coach for his son's soccer team and feels very proud of this decision.

SUMMARY

Alcohol and drug abuse is a pervasive problem in primary care and one that many health care providers would like to better detect and treat. Let's review the critical points covered in this chapter:

- In the contextual approach, substance-use problems are avoidance problems.

- The numbing effect of alcohol and drugs draws the patient out of present-moment awareness, often for long periods of time.

- Many patients benefit when you take an accepting, curious approach, which provides a model of acceptance and avoids triggering patient avoidance.

- You can move slowly and intentionally in helping these patients learn a variety of present-moment awareness strategies.

- Apart from the considerable health consequences of prolonged substance abuse, the toxic effect of addictive behavior is that it keeps patients out of contact with valued life directions and often causes harm to their loved ones.

- Getting patients to identify important personal values and to see substance use as a barrier to value-consistent action is a key principle in creating real behavior change in patients struggling with alcohol and drug use.

PREVIEW

In the next chapter, we will introduce you to a new approach to caring for patients with chronic pain.

CHAPTER 7

"Doc, This Pain Is Killing Me": Addressing Chronic Pain with Compassion

In separateness lies the world's great misery; in compassion lies the world's true strength.

—Buddha

A commonly accepted definition of chronic pain is pain that persists longer than the temporal course of natural healing associated with the particular type of injury or disease process the patient is experiencing. Psychological comorbidity is a frequent complication of chronic pain and one that complicates course and prognosis; for example, chronic pain significantly predicts onset of new depression, and depression significantly predicts onset of new chronic pain *and* other medical complaints (Tunks, Crook, & Weir, 2008). There also appears to be a significant overlap between post-traumatic stress disorder (PTSD) and chronic pain (Nampiaparampil, 2008).

Primary care management of chronic pain is difficult and frustrating, even for seasoned physicians. First, diagnosis is challenging, with imaging studies of chronic-pain patients often showing no discernible pathology or a level of damage that's far outstripped by the amount of pain the patient "should be" reporting. Second, patients who suffer from chronic pain often report simultaneous problems with frustration with medical providers (past and present) and fluctuating mood states that can (and often do) erupt during medical visits. The medical provider is thus faced with not only the task of addressing the mysteries of chronic pain, but also the active sense of mental suffering and discontent the patient brings to the clinic. Third, there's the omnipresent fear that you, the health care provider, are dealing with an addict who will misuse, abuse, or divert any prescribed pain medicines. Fourth, access to behavioral treatments is problematic, particularly for specialty multidisciplinary pain management programs. Even when patients access these services, their chronic pain is rarely completely relieved, and they return to their PCPs for ongoing management. These factors, together or in isolation, can create an atmosphere of mutual fear, distrust, and discouragement between the patient and provider.

Let's take a closer look at the issue of treating chronic pain with medications. While opioids and antidepressants (as well as other medications) may be useful, they are only a partial treatment at best, and it's difficult to find (and maintain) the delicate balance between beneficial effects and problematic side effects. With long-term use of opioids, patients may experience a loss of motivation and initiative, develop drug tolerance, and, in some cases, develop addiction. These problems, along with the problem of drug diversion, make medication management of chronic pain in primary care complex.

Before delving into behavioral strategies for PCPs, let's look briefly at psychological research findings pertinent to redesigning treatment of chronic pain in primary care. First, data from a variety of studies suggest the idea of a "pain gate" as a functional, rather than structural, aspect of the central nervous system. Factors like depression, anxiety, fear of pain, and a sedentary lifestyle, among others, stimulate opening of the pain gate, thereby increasing the patient's experience of pain. Additionally, patients with higher levels of pain show greater disruption of memory traces, suggesting they have deficits in working memory (Dick & Rashiq, 2007). With an understanding of the role of pain-gate–related vulnerabilities and the attention problems characteristic of patients with chronic pain, PCPs can better prepare to support real behavior change in this vulnerable group of patients.

Mindfulness exercises and value-based behavior-change strategies appear to help patients with chronic pain (McCracken & Eccleston, 2003; Dahl et al., 2004, Vowles et al., 2007). Before reading about this chapter's case example, consider three ideas that can supercharge your application of these approaches in primary care:

- Think of chronic pain as pain *and* the unwillingness to have it.

- Apply acceptance and value-based behavior-change principles to how you practice.

- Redirect your conversation with the patient with chronic pain from eliminating pain to accepting pain and living a meaningful life.

Encourage your patients to look closely at their goal or motivation concerning pain. Do they want to get rid of it, or do they want to learn to live a meaningful life, even with continued pain? Many times, chronic-pain patients will tell you that they want to be pain free. When you hear this, use workability questions: What have you done to be pain free? How has that worked in the short and long terms? Many times, patients say that what works in the short run (for example, pursuing larger dosages of analgesic medications) does not work in the long run (for example, does not reduce pain and instead brings new problems).

Remember that unwillingness to experience anything that's already present in our lives, including pain, brings additional suffering: the suffering of trying to avoid it, deny it, reason it away, or make someone else take responsibility for it.

Unwillingness in one person can easily bring out unwillingness in another, so finding ways to enhance your own willingness level is fundamental to improving your outcomes with chronic pain patients. A less-willing response to a patient who says, "This pain is killing me; I've got to have more medicine," might be, "No, I'm not going to give you an increase this month; you got one last month," or "Okay, but that's it; no higher dose after this." A more-willing response would sound more like, "I hear you; I know you are suffering, and I understand that you think medication will stop that suffering. Science says it won't. My saying this probably makes you uncomfortable, and admittedly, I feel uncomfortable too. My hope is that we can both accept our feelings of discomfort and keep talking." One of our favorite ways to remind ourselves to be present and model willingness is to maintain an awareness of our breath and our hands during the visit. Focus on slow diaphragmatic breathing and touch your fingertips together lightly, resting your hands in your lap. Keeping the hands soft somehow seems to help keep the conversation more compassionate. When we model willingness, we encourage a new conversation with the patient, a conversation about *acceptance*. Acceptance, rather than suppression or distraction, is the most powerful intervention for reducing the functional impairment associated with patients who have back pain (Vowles et al., 2007). Further, adding a component focused on the patient's values appears to augment acceptance interventions (Branstetter-Rost, Cushing, & Douleh, 2009).

With these guidelines in mind, let's turn our attention to the case of Ed and Dr. Andrews. As indicated in the following chapter-introduction box, we focus on three processes and demonstrate how to use four techniques in our case example. Since Ed is an established patient with a chronic problem, we do not demonstrate use of behavior-change interviewing tools in this chapter but instead briefly describe a pathway program for delivering ongoing care to patients with chronic pain. The Pain and Quality of Life (P&QOL) Pathway is a multidisciplinary, ACT-inspired program for the primary care setting that includes a monthly group visit. While not required, it's ideal to partner with a behavioral health (BH) provider when creating a pathway program. The primary care behavioral health (PCBH) model provides details about how to integrate behavioral health providers into primary care (see Robinson & Reiter, 2007, for more information).

Chronic Pain Interventions	
The Pain and Quality of Life Pathway	
Real Behavior Change Pocket Guide	
Process	**Technique**
Step Back from TEAMS and Unworkable Rules	TEAMS Sheet
Accept TEAMS and Focus on Action	Eagle Perspective
Connect with Values and Sustain Value-Consistent Action	▪ Bull's-Eye Worksheet (individual visit and group visit) ▪ All Hands on Deck (group visit)

Remember, when this symbol appears next to discussions about a diagram or worksheet, you can find a copy online at http://www .newharbingeronline.com/real-behavior-change-in-primary-care.html.

CASE EXAMPLE: ED AND DR. ANDREWS

Ed is a forty-five-year-old Native American with chronic back pain, arthritis in both knees, and chronic headaches. Dr. Andrews has been his doctor for the past five years. About a year ago, Dr. Andrews enrolled Ed in the clinic's Pain and Quality of Life (P&QOL) Pathway program, which requires him to attend monthly classes led by the clinic's behavioral health consultant (BHC), Dr. Wine.

Reason for Visit. Ed asks for an appointment to discuss back and knee pain and to discuss the possibility of changing pain medications.

Medical Status. Pain medications include a nonsteroidal anti-inflammatory drug (NSAID), amitriptyline, and a weak opioid. Ed is overweight and has diabetes; he takes oral diabetes medications.

Patient Concern. He needs more of his "hydrocodone or something stronger." He asks to see Dr. Andrews before going to the P&QOL class, so he can get "a prescription that works."

Patient's Life Context. Ed lives with his wife of twenty-two years, two of their adult children, and two grandchildren. Ed is a mural artist who is able to make a decent living by painting in local restaurants and homes. He supplements his work by selling fish he and his son catch during the fishing season. His wife works full-time as a clerk at a local casino. Ed loves his children and his wife. He has a brother who is an "alcoholic," but Ed doesn't "touch the sauce." He received training in mechanics during his four years in the military, but he injured his back at the end of the training and never actually worked as a mechanic. He takes two twenty-minute walks every day at the high-school track near his house, and he takes his diabetic medicines consistently. He also tests his blood sugars on a regular basis. He prefers fatty foods, but with his wife's support, he has taken to eating a salad almost every evening for dinner.

PLANNING AND PROVIDING TREATMENT

Because Dr. Andrews knows Ed well, we will bypass the demonstration of behavior-change interview tools demonstrated in the two previous chapters. For a new patient who suffers with chronic pain, use the Love, Work, Play, and Health Questions, and the Three-T and Workability Questions. Given that Ed is enrolled in the P&QOL Pathway, we begin with a brief description of this program, including the services provided by Dr. Wine, a psychologist who works with Dr. Andrews in this pathway.

Pain and Quality of Life Pathway

The Pain and Quality of Life (P&QOL) Pathway is a program that provides an ongoing approach to caring for primary care patients who have chronic pain. The PCP decides which patients to enroll in the program, and most often, patients selected for enrollment have long-standing problems with pain and are physically and psychologically dependent on pain medications. Many have additional medical problems, such as excess weight or even obesity, hypertension, cardiovascular problems, and diabetes. The P&QOL program saves you time, decreases unscheduled calls and visits, and facilitates appropriate medical care for comorbid medical problems that might otherwise be given short shrift with these patients due to the dominating nature of pain complaints. In addition, the pathway creates an opportunity to obtain monthly measures of patient functioning and provides patients with an opportunity to learn, apply, and evaluate behavioral interventions to improve quality of life. Patients receive medications at the end of the class, so no medical visit is required for prescribing. As the PCP, you may participate or even conduct the class, depending on your preference. A pain agreement specifies all elements of the P&QOL program, including class attendance, and patients sign the agreement at enrollment. Worksheet 7.1 describes providers' tasks in this multidisciplinary approach to primary care management of pain. Nurses may also help with this program by maintaining a registry of enrolled patients and working with the PCP regarding obtaining prescriptions during the week prior to the monthly class.

WORKSHEET 7.1
Pain and Quality of Life Pathway Activities for the Patient, PCP, and BHC Provider

Patient Activities	PCP Activities	BHC (or PCP) Activities
Request care for chronic pain	Enroll patient (provide description, assist patient with signing pain agreement, refer to BHC)	Host orientation visit with patient (describe class, respond to questions)
Follow pain agreement terms Attend classes Come to all medical and BH visits Respond promptly to request for urine analysis (UA) tests	Prescribe according to pain agreement terms Provide ongoing medical care Change treatment plan, as needed, and update pain agreement	Conduct monthly class (obtain objective data on patient functioning, teach behavioral strategies, work with RN in distributing pain medications, chart assessment results, and provide group interventions)

Ed's Visit with Dr. Andrews

Dr. Andrews started using the Bull's-Eye Worksheet with Ed when he enrolled in the P&QOL program a year ago. The plan supports continuity between Ed's care in individual visits with Dr. Andrews and in class visits with Dr. Wine.

ACCEPT TEAMS AND FOCUS ON ACTION

About six months ago, Dr. Andrews began supporting Ed's use of the eagle perspective when he read about it on a class-visit chart note. He asked Ed to describe it and learned that the eagle perspective was helping Ed improve his quality of life.

Eagle Perspective. This technique involves using the metaphor of a high-soaring eagle to describe a perspective that empowers humans to plan a course and stick with it, even in the presence of painful TEAMS. An eagle headed for a nest notices a rabbit here and there, feels the shift in the wind, and hears the screech of a red-tailed hawk, but continues to fly toward the nest. You might suggest that the patient simply take a deep breath and float up, letting go of both internal and external phenomena that distract her from continuing on her chosen course.

Ed first learned about eagle perspective in his monthly P&QOL class, when Dr. Wine talked about the perspective of a mouse and that of an eagle. A mouse looks at details, while an eagle sees the big picture. A mouse perspective on a pain sensation invites struggle, while an eagle perspective allows pain to be a smaller part of the picture and supports acceptance. Ed identifies with these ideas, because they are consistent with his Native American beliefs. He also likes to imagine being supported by eagle feathers in moving from mouse to eagle perspective, because eagle feathers are used in Native American healing practices. When he is able to remember to use the eagle perspective, he feels better able to take heart and gather the courage he needs to do what is most important to him.

DR. ANDREWS: Hello, Ed. I'm glad you came in today. Let's see, you have class at 3:00, right?

ED: Yes, I want you to change my prescription. I need something stronger or more pills. I've been out for a couple of days, and I'm in bad shape.

STEP BACK FROM TEAMS AND
UNWORKABLE RULES

Dr. Andrews uses a supportive technique called the TEAMS Sheet (review chapter 3), by letting himself and Ed step back from problematic TEAMS that sometimes come up during the course of their visits.

The TEAMS Sheet. In this technique, briefly explain each of the TEAMS elements and then ask the patient to use the TEAMS Sheet to identify negative TEAMS that tend to "push" her around. Ideally, you will ask the patient to use it in the visit when it's introduced and then to practice sitting down and filling out the sheet at home for a few minutes every day. At the end of the brief home-practice periods, the patient can jot down a few notes about the TEAMS she observed, bringing back the results at follow-up. Once the patient learns to use the TEAMS Sheet, you and the patient can use the sheet during visits, particularly when interaction between you and the patient may be under the influence of negative TEAMS that limit both of you in experiencing the present moment during the visit. Dr. Andrews responds affirmatively to Ed's request for more medicine but requests that they use the TEAMS Sheet and sit in silent observance for the first two to three minutes of the visit.

DR. ANDREWS: Okay, I hear you, but let's get off to a good start. Remember the way we started our last visit by sitting quietly and just trying to be present for a minute or two? Remember how we tried to notice our thoughts, emotions, associations, memories, and sensations, and accept them as we sat in silence? I would like to do that now. To help us remember what we are trying to notice in our minds as we sit together, I have this reminder for each of us *[hands Ed the TEAMS Sheet in worksheet 7.2 and models holding a second copy in his lap].*

ED   *[looking at the TEAMS sheet]:* Okay, you're the doc. I'll play your game.

WORKSHEET 7.2 TEAMS SHEET

In my mind, I see and make room for:				
Thoughts	Emotions	Associations	Memories	Sensations

Ed and Dr. Andrews sit together in silence, both distracted by noises in the hallway and their own TEAMS. However, as their eyes meet, there's a growing sense of connection. Dr. Andrews calls time at three minutes and then requests that both he and Ed use as few words as possible to speak, focusing on the most important things to say. He asks Ed to go first.

ED: I'm embarrassed and upset. I am a proud man and don't want to beg for pills. I want to be strong for my family.

DR. ANDREWS: I feel sad. I want to help you. I think pills look like a gift but don't have substance.

ED: I want help; I've been grouchy at home.

DR. ANDREWS: I'm trying to use the eagle perspective right now, and I keep being drawn to the thought, *I have to make your pain go away.*

ED [smiling]: I get stuck on that too.

DR. ANDREWS: Ed, I'll increase your prescription by five pills a month, but we know that's not the magic. The magic is the work you do in the class and the ways you apply it in your life, like when you taught your granddaughter about eagle perspective.

ED [smiling]: I think I need to make one of these [holding up the TEAMS Sheet] to use at home when I start to get wound up about the pain.

DR. ANDREWS: You can have that one, Ed. It occurs to me that when
you have the urge to use more of the medicine than
prescribed, you can try just sitting with your TEAMS
Sheet for five minutes. It might help. Will you give it a
try?

ED: Yes, Dr. Andrews, I will.

Dr. Andrews ends the visit by writing a few notes on a Bull's-Eye
Worksheet (see sample worksheet 7.3) and giving Ed a copy of the work-
sheet and the TEAMS Sheet. He wants to support Ed in stepping back from
TEAMS and unworkable rules at home.

SAMPLE WORKSHEET 7.3
Ed's Bull's-Eye Worksheet (from Dr. Andrews)

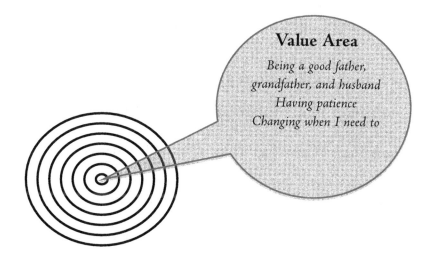

Value Area

*Being a good father,
grandfather, and husband
Having patience
Changing when I need to*

Action Step(s):

1. *Sit quietly, holding TEAMS Sheet when stressed about pain and medicines.*

2. *Use eagle perspective.*

Ed's Visit to the Pain and Quality of Life Class

Sample worksheet 7.4 summarizes the agenda Dr. Wine follows in the P&QOL class. Using a consistent agenda helps her to be efficient and encourages class members to develop group cohesion over time. Total class time is approximately one hour. The class begins with introductions and cohesion-building activities, and it ends with commitment to value-based behavior-change plans developed in the group. The BH provider maintains a packet of materials for each class member, distributes it at the beginning of the class, and collects it at class conclusion. Member packets include quality-of-life assessment questions, a summary sheet for assessment findings during the calendar year, and bull's-eye worksheets. Class members sign in on a prescription request sheet fifteen minutes after the start of class. The nurse working with the BH provider uses this list to prepare for distribution of prescriptions at the end of class (or to arrange to have prescriptions filled during the class for patients using the onsite pharmacy).

SAMPLE WORKSHEET 7.4
Pain and Quality of Life Class Agenda

Time	BH Provider Tasks	Class Member Tasks
0–5 minutes	Pass out packets to class members. Facilitate introductions (when new members are present). Ask about birthdays in the past month and lead "Happy Birthday to You."	Introduce self. Notice urges to talk about pain. Show respect to others present.

5–10 minutes	Conduct brief lecture (if new patients are present), including goals regarding pain (acceptance vs. avoidance), workability of control and avoidance agendas. Introduce bull's-eye.	Listen. For advanced class members, participate in teaching.
10–15 minutes	Ask quality-of-life questions.	Respond in writing to questions. Sign in on prescription sheet.
15–25 minutes	Conduct one-to-two minute, one-on-one check-ins with members, comparing current scores with the previous month's and noting any concerns indicating a need for a medical visit.	Work alone or with a partner (patient choice) on Bull's-Eye Worksheet. Reflect on impact of plan from previous month, clarifying value statements, and plan behavior change for coming month.
25–35 minutes	Lead discussion concerning member experiences with Bull's-Eye Worksheet and use of previously introduced strategies to improve QOL.	Participate.
35–45 minutes	Teach new skill, conduct experiential activity, or both.	Participate.
45–55 minutes	Introduce the All Hands on Deck game.	Participate.
55–60 minutes	Ask each patient to stand, if able, and share his or her plan for the coming month in thirty seconds.	State your plan for the coming month.

During class, Ed discusses his plan for the previous month with Tom, a classmate. Tom started the program shortly after Ed. They often sit next to each other, and Ed looks forward to talking with Tom. Ed had planned to explore attending a whittling group, because he has more problems with knee and back pain when he works on murals, particularly larger ones. He thought he might be able to make some money selling carvings for the Native American museum gift shop. His father taught him to work with wood when he was younger, and he felt he had some talent for it. In talking with Tom, Ed decides his not following through on taking the whittling class was from letting his "bad mood get in the way"; he got distracted and didn't follow through on the plan. They talk briefly about Ed's values concerning carving. He knows he wants to provide for his family and be independent, and he realizes while talking with Tom that he also sees carving as a way to express his creativity and spirituality. In his brief one-on-one check-in with Dr. Wine, she points out that Ed's quality-of-life scores haven't gone down, even though he had more problems with pain, depression, and grumpiness during the month. Her words of encouragement feel good to Ed.

All Hands on Deck. At every group visit, one or two people have an opportunity to play the All Hands on Deck game. Because Dr. Wine's instruction goes a little long, there is time for only one class member to be the ship's captain, and Ed asks to steer the ship. In this game, the captain states where he wants the ship to go. The target location is usually chosen for how well it represents a destination for a value-consistent action. Ed wants to explore new ways to make a living, and exploring carving is a step in that direction. After stating the destination (for example, attending a whittling class), the captain recruits four or five class members to be the ship's crew. The role of each crew member is to represent a specific barrier that the captain believes would distract or even derail his efforts to sail to the destination. Ed has clear ideas about his TEAMS elements, and he relates them to five volunteers from the group.

THOUGHTS: I don't have the energy; life has sucked it out of me.

EMOTIONS: Sadness, bitterness

ASSOCIATIONS: Vague association of self-worth relying on ability to provide for family

MEMORIES: Injury in the military, future he wanted

SENSATIONS: Pain all over

Each crew member writes a few words to serve as reminders of what to say to Ed as he attempts to steer the ship. Ed and his crew walk to the front of the room. Ed takes the imaginary helm and shouts, "All hands on deck!" The crew lines up around him, ready to help out. Ed says, "Here I go. I want to find a new way to make money to take care of myself and my family. I'm going to the carving group." Knowing the rules of the game, the crew members start to circle around Ed in an attempted mutiny, each saying something related to his assigned TEAMS element: "You're broken. You're worn out. You have pain all over your body. Life has chewed you up and spit you out." Ed feels the urge to argue, to defend himself. He is able to accept that urge and gives only a nod of acknowledgment as the crew members pass him by. He stays at the helm, with his eyes on his destination for four minutes, and Dr. Wine calls time. She asks Ed to give a brief summary of his experience, and he simply responds, "I'm learning." Dr. Wine thanks Ed for his courage and thanks his crew for being helpful classmates.

Bull's-Eye Worksheet. When Ed updates his Bull's-Eye Worksheet in class, he includes practicing the eagle perspective during the first five minutes of his morning walk (see sample worksheet 7.5). He also underlines the plan he made the previous month to go to the whittling group. At the end of the group, he stands proudly as he looks down at his plan and reads to his classmates, "I will go to the whittling group next month," and he knows he will.

SAMPLE WORKSHEET 7.5
Ed's Bull's-Eye Worksheet
(from the P&QOL Class)

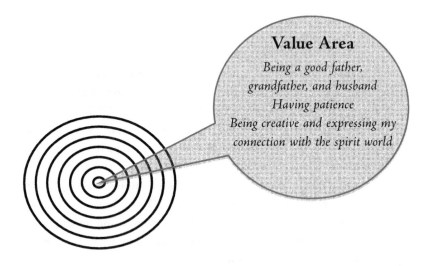

Value Area

Being a good father,
grandfather, and husband
Having patience
Being creative and expressing my
connection with the spirit world

Action Step(s):

1. *Use eagle perspective every morning for the first five minutes of my morning walk.*

2. *I will go to the whittling group next month.*

SUMMARY

This chapter was jam-packed with ideas for improving outcomes with chronic-pain patients. While our case example involved the presence of a behavioral health provider working as a primary care team member, a PCP and nurse team alone can use most of these ideas. Let's review the specifics:

- Define chronic pain as pain *and* the unwillingness to have it, which gives you and the patient an opportunity to look at the costs of struggling against pain and to shift the focus of your work to improving the patient's quality of life.

- Unwillingness in one person can bring out unwillingness in another, which brings us to the second direction we encourage you to explore in working with patients with chronic pain: find ways to enhance your willingness level so that you can better model acceptance.

- Teaching acceptance techniques, in combination with value-based behavior-change strategies, is powerful medicine for patients with chronic pain. While not used in the case example in this chapter, the Three (or Five) Senses and Balloon Breath exercises often help patients with chronic pain improve attention and reduce tension.

- Chronic-pain patients respond well to metaphors, such as eagle perspective and bull's-eye planning and, in a class context, physical metaphors, like the All Hands on Deck metaphor.

- We encourage you to read more about the primary care behavioral health model (Robinson & Reiter, 2007) and partner with a behavioral health provider who will work with you as a primary care team member to improve outcomes for the growing number of patients who are challenged by this very difficult problem.

PREVIEW

In the next chapter, you will learn to apply ACT to another high-impact group of primary care patients. Patients with symptoms of anxiety and depression are a large and growing group of patients.

CHAPTER 8

A Fresh Approach to the Daily Duo: Anxiety and Depression

Christopher Robin to Pooh: Promise me you'll always remember—you're braver than you believe and stronger than you seem and smarter than you think.

—A. A. Milne

For years, people went to their doctors and other health care providers to hear words of encouragement, and they received them, took heart, and continued to work with the difficult hand life had dealt them. Then, a new perspective on suffering evolved based on the notion that suffering was a brain problem, the result of a chemical imbalance. Even though the science for this story was weak at best, powerful pharmaceutical companies supported it. During the 1990s, these companies attained the right to directly market antianxiety, antidepressant, and sleep medications to potential customers. Their television ads were (and are currently!) potent, and misleading. Many people became convinced by their message and sought medication for their "illnesses." In a large study of primary care patients, half of those prescribed antidepressants for depression did not qualify for any diagnosis of depression (Katon et al., 1996). Many primary care patients are psychologically dependent on using medications to help control undesirable mood states, even though these medicines may have limited benefit at best. For example, a recent meta-analysis of all drug-company-sponsored clinical trials suggested that antidepressants are not significantly more effective than placebo medicine (Turner, Mathews, Linardatos, Tell, & Rosenthal, 2008)! These facts notwithstanding, primary care providers have the dubious distinction of prescribing more antidepressant (and anxiolytic) medications than any other health profession, including psychiatry (Beardsley, Gardocki, Larson, & Hidalgo, 1988).

However, the pendulum is swinging back now, and we see increasing efforts to provide behavioral interventions (and encouragement) in primary care settings. Mindfulness, acceptance, and value-based behavior-change interventions are practical and effective for depressed primary care patients (Katon et al., 1996; Robinson, Wischman, & del Vento, 1996). These interventions can be delivered in brief primary care visits and supported phone visits with nursing staff (Meresman et al., 2003). Additional resources suggest that contextual behavior-change interventions may be effective in groups guided by available books (see for example Strosahl & Robinson, 2008, for a curriculum for a depression class; Forsyth & Eifert, 2007, for a curriculum for an anxiety class).

This is very good news because, considered together, depression and anxiety are more prevalent than the most common chronic diseases. In a worldwide study of 25,000 consecutive adults screened in 150 sites in 14 countries, the most common mental disorders were depressive disorders (11.7 percent) and anxiety disorders (9 percent), with 4.6 percent of the patients reporting both (Sartorius, Ustün, Lecrubier, & Wittchen, 1996). More recent findings suggest that 18 percent of people in America will suffer from an anxiety disorder every year (Kessler et al., 2005). The vast majority of these patients will be treated by a primary care provider and will never see a mental health specialist (Wang et al., 2005). Depression, if expanded to include chronic low-grade depression (often called "minor depression"), is even more prevalent than anxiety in primary care. Primary care patients over age 65 are of particular concern, because around 10 percent have clinically significant symptoms of depression, and depression is often undetected in older patients, particularly men (Unützer, 2007).

The ever-increasing financial impact of mood-related problems in primary care is a result of exploding pharmaceutical costs and the increased medical costs of providing care. For example, patients with symptoms of anxiety (for example, dizziness, tinnitus, gastrointestinal distress) tend to receive more expensive diagnostic procedures than nonanxious patients (Katon, Roy-Byrne, Russo, & Cowley, 2002). Another important thing to remember is that the long-term functional impact of mood disorders is greater than the impact of many chronic diseases like diabetes, congestive heart failure, angina, and arthritis (Wells et al., 1989).

Given the prevalence and impact of mood problems in primary care, the United States Preventive Services Task Force (2009) has addressed the practice of screening adults for depression in primary care. It recommends screening contingent on the ability to provide timely treatment and closely monitored follow-up care for such patients. In other words, it doesn't help to screen for depression or anxiety if you don't offer the patient an effective treatment. To help you develop an effective way of addressing depression and anxiety, we will teach you a contextual approach to these problems that will complement any traditional medication treatments you might elect to use.

Think of anxiety and depression as sitting on opposite ends of a single continuum. At one end are patients who predominately experience depression, and at the other end are patients who predominately experience anxiety. The reason we look at mood problems this way is because the same ACT processes are at work, only in different ways. Depressed patients tend to live more in the past (and focus on past failures and disappointments), while anxious patients focus on the future (and often anticipate the worst). For example, a patient who experiences depression after a job loss may have TEAMS like *I've done everything I could again, and nothing works out for me. I try to do the same things other people do—work hard and all that—but in the end I lose, and there's really no one there for me.* While women tend to report sadness, men may be more likely to report irritability or anger. Depressed patients may experience associations of being alone and unprotected, in their current experience and also perhaps as children. Memories tend to be focused on shortcomings or mistreatments in the family, school, and work contexts. Sensations often include fatigue, headache, and feeling "gassed." Patients prone to responding to stress with symptoms of depression tend to lack skills for stepping back from painful TEAMS and limiting self-stories. They often have dearly held values and cry when you ask them to talk about them. Rather than experience the pain in accepting the discrepancy between what they want their lives to be about and what they are at present, they use a variety of coping strategies to numb themselves (such as overeating, watching television, using drugs and alcohol, using increased doses of psychotropic medications). Remember that depression is not sadness or anger; it's more akin to absence of feeling, which explains many of the seminal symptoms of depression: disinterest, fatigue, concentration problems, and so on.

Anxious patients, on the other hand, focus on the future, often anticipating the worst. For example, let's think through a medical student's experience of test anxiety. This patient may have TEAMS like *I'm smart, but if I get anxious during this test, there's no way I'll be able to complete it. I've studied a lot and shouldn't even be sweating this, but I am, and I can't seem to control it. If I blow this test, my parents will think I'm a big loser. This is ridiculous.* Corresponding emotions might include fear, apprehension, and frustration. Associations might include *trying, but coming up short.* Memories might include coming home with B's and one C in the seventh grade, and being grounded by parents who scolded, "We are not average in this family, and you are not going to change our standard." Sensations might include chest pain or pressure, a lump in the throat, shortness of breath, light-headedness, trembling, dizziness, flushing or a sense of increased body temperature, a sense of rapid heartbeat, or some combination. As you can see in this example, the patient with anxiety overidentifies with the mind's catastrophic predictions. In addition, the anxious patient avoids directly experiencing the feelings triggered by images of the future and the past. Just as depression is an attempt to avoid sadness, loss, or anger, anxiety is also an attempt to avoid unpleasant TEAMS, particularly fear—of failure, disappointing others, abandonment, health problems, and so on. Although the TEAMS themes and unworkable rules that predominate in depression and anxiety differ, the net results are difficulties staying present, emotional pain, troubling images and memories, and physical discomforts. Having swallowed a negative self-story, a person's ability to set a meaningful life course and pursue it with consistency is limited.

One final thing to remember is that in the center of the mood continuum, you will see patients who have a mixture of anxiety and depression. Indeed, you can think of this continuum as a dynamic process. Some patients who present with depression may have struggled for years to control their anxiety and eventually fell into a deep depression because their anxiety is "uncontrollable." Similarly, patients with a primary history of depression may gradually develop severe anxiety because of their inability to control their depression and their tendency to worry and to anticipate a negative future.

For now, let's consider the case of Bella and look at how Dr. Soto, her family physician, uses behavior-change tools to improve Bella's quality of life—and mood. As indicated in the following chapter-introduction box, we focus on three processes and demonstrate how to use four techniques in our case example. After the case example, we will briefly introduce the Living Life Well class, which can help patients with strong habit histories to learn new ways of coping with stress.

Anxiety and Depression Interventions

Three-T and Workability Questions

Core Process Assessment Tool (CPAT)

Real Behavior Change Pocket Guide

Process	Technique
Step Back from TEAMS and Unworkable Rules	TEAMS Sheet
Experience the Present Moment	▪ Three (or Five) Senses ▪ Time Line
Use Observer Self to See Limiting Self-Stories	▪ Circles of Self ▪ Miracle Question
The Living Life Well Class	

Remember, when this symbol appears next to discussions about a diagram or worksheet, you can find a copy online at http://www.newharbingeronline.com/real-behavior-change-in-primary-care.html.

CASE EXAMPLE: BELLA AND DR. SOTO

Bella is a sixty-five-year-old recent widow who retired from teaching. Dr. Soto has been her doctor for the past seven years.

Reason for Visit. Bella came to the clinic for a planned visit concerning sleep problems and ongoing problems with fatigue.

Medical Status. Bella has hyperlipidemia and high blood pressure; she takes medications for both conditions. She is slightly overweight.

Patient Concern. Bella wants to "feel better."

Patient's Life Context. Bella lives alone in an apartment near her church. She moved there two years ago after her husband of forty years died and she sold their home. After retiring from teaching elementary school at age sixty, she had volunteered at the library, but gave this up when her husband became ill. Randall, her husband, struggled for several years with cancer, and Bella cared for him fastidiously. She takes pride in having helped him to die at home, but Dr. Soto saw the price Bella paid during this difficult time and worries about her recovery. While Bella continues to take her medicines and has moved to a more easily managed living situation, she seems to have "pulled back" from life since her retirement, and she now seems distant and distracted during medical visits. She rarely sees her two sons, who live out of town, and even though she lives within walking distance of her church, she rarely attends services anymore. During his medical visits with Bella, Dr. Soto asks questions to help him better understand Bella's TEAMS experience. Sample worksheet 8.1 summarizes what he has heard in recent visits.

SAMPLE WORKSHEET 8.1
Bella's TEAMS

Thoughts	*Life just isn't the same for me. Randall was my best friend and my husband. I try not to think of him or what happened. It just seems like everything I do is just going through the motions. Nothing really interests me anymore. My sons don't seem to care about how I'm doing. They don't call, and I don't call; I don't want to be a bother.*
Emotions	Sadness, loss, loneliness, boredom
Associations	*Being alone is like being of little value or no value.*
Memories	Remembering the moments before Randall died, the pain of saying good-bye
Sensations	Fatigue, chest pain, burning eyes, neckache, and backache

Behavior-Change Interview

Dr. Soto uses the Three-T and Workability Questions to help him understand Bella's request for help with "feeling better." To help him understand more specifically what Bella meant when she said she wanted to feel better, he asks, "What bothers you most about the way you feel now?" Bella responds, "Feeling tired out and not sleeping well." He focuses on these problems in the Three-T and Workability Questions, and sample worksheet 8.2 summarizes the results.

SAMPLE WORKSHEET 8.2
Bella's Responses to the Three-T and Workability Questions

Area	Questions	Patient Responses
Time	When did your sleep and energy problems start?	Long ago, maybe four or five years, when Randall fell ill. I was nervous a lot and missed out on sleep when he was sick at night. I think feeling tired just started to feel normal to me, but now I just don't get much of anything done.
Triggers	Can you identify anything that sets off a bad night of sleep or a bad day energy-wise?	Well, things are worse when I am thinking about how my life isn't what I wanted, that my sons live far away and that I'm a widow and (begins to tear up)—I try not to think these things. There's no point in self-pity.
	How about things that start a better day or night cycle?	I think I probably sleep better when I take a walk in the morning, and maybe I do feel more motivated when I get back home, but most days I feel too tired to go out.
Trajectory	Over the course of the past five years, has your quality of sleep and your energy level varied—that is, been better at times, worse at other times?	I think I slept better when I lived in my old house; I kind of had my family, my memories, around me. I also slept a little better when my sister came to visit me last fall. We played dominoes at night and enjoyed each other's company. She got me out walking, too.

Workability Questions	What have you tried to cope with this problem? How have these strategies worked over time? Are you getting the kind of results you want?	Counting sheep, but that doesn't really work. I just end up tossing and turning and thinking about how tired I'll be tomorrow.

Dr. Soto summarizes information from the Three-T and Workability Questions in this way: "So, let's see if I get it. You've been having trouble with sleeping and feeling tired since Randall became ill four or five years ago. You try to not think about missing Randall and how your boys live far away, and you hope that if you can avoid that, you'll be okay. But that isn't working in the sense of helping you feel better. You count sheep, and that doesn't help you sleep. What does seem to help is going for walks, being with people like your sister, and doing fun things, like playing dominoes. Is that a good summary?"

Planning and Providing Treatment

To plan interventions and track progress, Dr. Soto uses the CPAT to conceptualize Bella's relative strengths and weaknesses. Bella seems to be living in the past a lot of the time and seems to expend her energy on avoiding ever-present painful memories. She also seems to be buying into a story that limits her expression of her values at this point; she valued being a mother and wife, but with her husband's death and her sons' emancipation, her story leaves her with nowhere to go. Given his long-term relationship with Bella, Dr. Soto knows firsthand about her values and her ability to persist in chosen directions. He decides to focus first on helping her better experience the present moment. If she can live a little more in the "now," she will probably be better able to accept the pain of loss and change and to tap into her observer self to see how her self-story limits her.

SAMPLE WORKSHEET 8.3
Bella's Core Process Assessment Tool (CPAT)

Six Core Processes: Psychological Rigidity	Patient Rating Today	Six Core Processes: Psychological Flexibility
Lives in the past or future	__X_____	Experiences the present moment
Disconnected from values	_____X__	Strongly connected with values
Engages in impulsive, self-defeating action or inaction	_____X__	Sustains value-consistent action
Stuck in limiting self-stories	_____X_____	Uses observer self to see limiting self-stories
Stuck in TEAMS and unworkable rules	_____X_____	Steps back from TEAMS and unworkable rules
Actively avoids TEAMS	__X_____	Accepts TEAMS and focuses on action

EXPERIENCE THE PRESENT MOMENT

Recalling that Bella has been a gardener, Dr. Soto asks her about her ability to experience elements of nature when she does manage to get out of the house to take a walk. He asks, "Do you notice variations in the color of green, see little buds, hear birds sing, or smell fresh-cut grass?" Bella responds that she does at times and that these sensations do please her. Dr. Soto then asks her to do an experiment with him to see how she can use her senses to be present anytime, even indoors.

Three (or Five) Senses. In this exercise, as the PCP, you ask the patient to notice three (or five) present-moment experiences using each of the five senses. The following dialogue illustrates how Dr. Soto uses this technique with Bella.

DR. SOTO: Let's have you start by exhaling completely and then
             allowing air to flow into your chest. Try that several times,
             tuning in to the rise and fall of your chest, and the feeling
             of air entering your nose and then leaving your nose. You
             might even notice that the air is warmer when you exhale.
             There, you are already experiencing more of the present
             moment. Next, I want you to tune in to your ears and your
             ability to hear. Distinguish a sound and name it aloud.

BELLA: I hear a motor running, maybe a machine of some kind.

DR. SOTO: Yes, now listen for another.

BELLA: I hear footsteps and people talking, but I can't make out
             what they are saying.

DR. SOTO: Great. Now, I want you to focus on your sense of touch.
             Name two things you feel at this very moment.

BELLA: I feel my fingertips touching—and I feel my legs touch the
             chair. Hmm, I can feel where my glasses rest on my nose.

DR. SOTO: You're pretty good at this. Let's see how it goes with your
             using a few more of your senses.

Dr. Soto continues to walk Bella through her present-moment sensory experiences. Then, he provides information about why reconnecting with these skills might be helpful to her at this point in time.

DR. SOTO: The more often you are able to be in the present moment,
             the better able you will be to make fresh choices and to
             learn from your experience. When we go through a bad spell
             in our lives—lots of change and losing loved ones—we often
             pull back from life. While that might help temporarily, it
             can become a habit, and we can lose our perspective and just
             stay in that hunkered-down kind of position.

Dr. Soto asks Bella to take daily walks and to practice using her five senses during her walks. He also wants to help Bella gain some flexibility in her perspective on life. At a follow-up visit, he may use the Time Line exercise (see chapter 3) to help her further develop skills for experiencing the present moment.

Time Line. This technique involves teaching the patient to follow TEAMS by moving her finger up and down a horizontal line (imagined or drawn on paper). Dr. Soto will teach Bella to move her finger to the left side when memories (for example, saying goodbye to her husband) show up. When she is thinking about the future ("If I go to church no one will greet me"), she notices this and moves her finger to the right side of the line. Dr. Soto can link this skill practice to the Three Senses exercise by saying something like "The middle of the line is the present moment, like when you smell a flower or see ping show up in a sunset."

USE OBSERVER SELF TO SEE LIMITING SELF-STORIES

Dr. Soto decides to take a few more minutes to jump-start Bella's ability to shift from ruminating about the past and worrying about the future to being focused in the present moment so that she is better able to consider ways to improve her life. Toward this end, he uses the Miracle Question, an interview technique often used in solution-focused interviewing (de Shazer, 1988).

Miracle Question. This question, first suggested by developers of solution-focused brief therapy, is quite useful in helping patients defuse and consider a more open perspective. The question may be phrased in a variety of ways, some examples of which follow.

Example 1: Let's pretend that you go to bed tonight, and while you are sleeping, a miracle happens. You don't know what has happened, but when you awaken in the morning, various things in your life have changed. You notice them as you go through the day. What do you notice first? What's different?

Example 2: Let's pretend for a moment that I have a magic wand that I can wave to help you feel better instantly. What's different about you? What do I see that tells me you feel better?

Example 3: If a miracle happened, and you suddenly felt better, how would your life be different?

Bella responds well to this question, explaining that she would be going for walks, attending church, perhaps going back to the library to volunteer one morning a week, and maybe planning a visit with her sister. Dr. Soto smiles and says he hopes she will surprise him by trying one of those changes before their next visit in two weeks. On the action steps section of the Bull's-Eye Worksheet, he notes her plan to take walks using her five senses, and he simply writes the word "Miracle" above the behavior changes she plans to make. He gives it to her as a reminder of what they discussed during this visit.

Providing Follow-Up Care for Bella

Bella returns for follow-up in two weeks. She smiles when Dr. Soto comes into the room, and she begins to tell him about her walks and what she noticed on them. She has met several people in her neighborhood and has talked with her sister about a visit. She also attended church and felt welcomed by a variety of people there.

USE OBSERVER SELF TO SEE LIMITING SELF-STORIES

Dr. Soto hopes to help Bella strengthen her observer self so she can have a larger perspective on her story about her life as presented and move beyond it.

Circles of Self. Dr. Soto draws three circles on the exam-room table paper (see worksheet 8.4), then asks Bella to do an exercise with him.

WORKSHEET 8.4 CIRCLES OF SELF

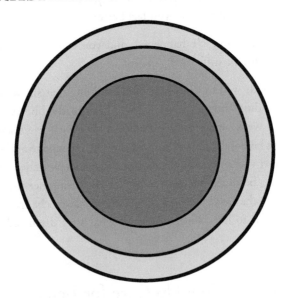

DR. SOTO: This exercise is called Circles of Self. Imagine three ways of looking at yourself, with each represented by a circle. Let's have the inner circle be the stories you tell about yourself, the way you'd describe yourself to someone you are just getting to know. What might you say?

BELLA: Well, I'd say I'm sixty-five years old, a widow, and a mother of two boys, and that I live alone, like to read, go for walks, and play dominoes and board games.

DR. SOTO: Right. And then you have stories that you might tell someone who knew you well—for example, me. These would go in that circle too. For instance, what might you say to me about who you are?

BELLA: Well, mostly I want you to think well of me, but I can tell you things like "I'm disappointed in myself" or "I've been feeling sorry for myself."

DR. SOTO: Okay, good. We all have stories like this about ourselves, and when we tell them, we tend to believe them 100 percent.

When we believe them 100 percent, there's not much room left for us to see other possible perspectives, so we need to develop skills that help us shift to the next circle. That second circle is where we have more present-moment sensory experiences, as you've been having on your walks. You can stay focused on present-moment experiences even while you are aware that your mind is telling stories about who you are. When you are better able to experience things in the present-moment circle, you are better able to choose what you do and are more independent of your life stories. Is this making sense to you, Bella?

BELLA: Yes, I think so. You're saying that when I feel sad and think I'm all alone in the world, I can just think that and feel that, but I can still go out and use my senses to experience the world. Right?

DR. SOTO: Yes, and that brings me to the third circle, and notice that this circle is way bigger than the story circle and takes in the present-moment senses circle. The simplest way to think about this circle is to imagine that there's an ongoing conversation in your mind. The speaker is your mind. It can speak to you about stories, or it can report back to you on second-by-second experiences you are having, such as when you are walking or working in your garden. Think of this biggest circle, here, as the you that listens and observes. This part of yourself has been listening and watching the conversation in your mind since you were a very young child. There has always been a "you" that listens and that has never changed across your life, even though you have had many, many life experiences, your body has changed, and your beliefs have changed. The one part of you that doesn't change is the you that's there to listen. Sometimes people call this your observing self or witnessing self. It's a place where you can see your whole life in perspective, where you can feel compassion for your struggles and those of others. It's a place where your wisdom, intuition, and inspiration all live. This part of yourself is a sanctuary you can enter whenever you are being pushed around by negative stories or when you are having trouble just staying present in your life. Are you following me?

BELLA: I understand what you are saying, even though it's hard to say so with words.

DR. SOTO: This is a part of yourself that's always present, and it takes some practice to learn how to enter into it. Doing things like walking and just noticing everything around you is one way to move into observing-self mode. Another way is to practice breathing quietly and just holding still, even if your mind is busy with stories. Is there something you would like to add to your lifestyle that might help you connect daily with this "observing self" part of you?

BELLA: I could take five to ten minutes each morning when I wake up to just breathe slowly and regularly, and "watch my mind," as you say. I used to pray in the morning when I was younger, and I remember how peaceful I felt afterward.

The Living Life Well Class

The Living Life Well class is a seven-session series that can support skill development among patients struggling with various symptoms of anxiety and depression. The curriculum was tested in brief visits with depressed primary care patients, and it was found to improve patient skills and symptoms of depression more than usual primary care (Katon et al., 1996). Materials for delivering this one-hour class are available in *Living Life Well: New Strategies for Hard Times* (Robinson, 1996). A PCP or a behavioral health provider (who partners with a PCP or group of PCPs) can teach or co-teach the class. It's important that the class be highly accessible, so that any patient may come to any class at any time without obligation to come to other classes. Toward this goal of open access (and to help you better address the high prevalence of depression and anxiety among your patients), we recommend placing posters in your clinic announcing the class topics and planned dates. The following table shows an example of a Living Life Well class poster.

Living Life Well Classes with Dr. Soto on Mondays, 4:00–5:00 p.m.

Date	Class Name	Topic
May 1	The Basics of Behavior Change: Hoping, Planning and Doing	Learn the basics of living the way you want to
May 8	How to Accept Difficulties and Pursue Your Values	Learn to choose to do what's most important (even when it's very difficult)
May 15	Caring for Your Body-Mind	Learn how to create sensations of wellness
May 22	Dealing with Conflicts	Learn how to say what you want and to have healthy disagreements
May 29	Expressing Yourself Well	Learn how to let go and "not do," and to pursue more of your creative potential
June 5	Planning Your Lifestyle	Learn to make healthy choices and to persevere

SUMMARY

Congratulations! You've completed a chapter that can help you provide better care to a very large group of patients. Let's review the key points:

■ Depression and anxiety exist on a single continuum supported by TEAMS avoidance, inability to stay in the present moment, and lack of perspective taking on negative self-stories.

- Remember that patients with mild symptoms of depression and anxiety are at risk of being overtreated with medications; they might benefit more from behavioral interventions and support.

- Avoid confusing collections of psychological symptoms or syndromes with disease conditions.

- Normalize patient symptoms by linking them to specific life stresses.

- Help patients develop present-moment skills by using interventions such as the Three (or Five) Senses exercise.

- Help patients learn to shift perspectives. Depression's *I'm a loser* and anxiety's *I'm in danger* perspectives are just perspectives on the self and the world. We can help our patients see these stories from the observer-self perspective, where acceptance and value-consistent action are more likely.

PREVIEW

In the next chapter, you will learn to apply ACT to patients with histories of trauma.

CHAPTER 9

Living in the Past,
Dying in the Present:
Trauma and Violence

For the majority of us, the past is a regret, the future an experiment.

—Mark Twain

There's a good reason this is the longest chapter of this part dealing with the most common clinical problems encountered in medical practice. Trauma and the violence that precedes it are the "nuclear fuel" that promotes suffering and a loss of vital living on an almost unimaginable scale. Most patients with long-term problems with social adjustment, chronic mood disorders, or drug and alcohol problems have trauma histories, often dating back to childhood and adolescence, and are often retraumatized as adults.

As medical providers, we tend to underestimate the prevalence and impact of violence and trauma on the health status of our patients. In 2007, 5,177,130 crimes of violence were committed in the United States (Bureau of Justice Statistics, 2007). Victims of violence crowd the waiting rooms in emergency departments and in primary care. Sadly, the majority of violent crimes are between family members (McCaig & Burt, 2004). Victims of violence and abuse are twice as likely to use health care services and are twice as expensive to treat on an annual basis, but they typically do not link their somatic complaints to past victimization (Koss, Koss, & Woodruff, 1991; Walker et. al., 2003). Victimization is also associated with a lowered health-related quality of life (Conway, Hu, Warshaw, Kim, & Bullon, 1995). The prevalence of one common sequela of victimization, post-traumatic stress disorder (PTSD), is estimated to be between 6.8 and 12.3 percent in the United States adult population (Kessler et. al., 2005); one study showed that 65 percent of patients in a community-clinic sample reported exposure to victimization and trauma, with a subsequent PTSD rate of 12 percent (Stein, McQuaid, Pedrelli, Lenox, & McCahill, 2000). Women are ten times more likely to be raped or molested than men, and four times more likely to develop PTSD than men after controlling for exposure to traumatic events (Vieweg et al., 2006).

This astounding set of research findings also suggests why it's often difficult for primary care providers to help patients who have been victimized. First, they tend to present with physical complaints that mask their underlying issues. The provider can easily get caught in a cycle of symptom chasing that keeps the discussion from focusing on underlying issues. Second, the humiliation, stigma, shame, guilt, and self-loathing that are part of the normal emotional aftermath of victimization make it difficult for such patients to ask for help with their emotional pain. The main question this chapter addresses is how can you, as a PCP, better identify patients with trauma-related symptoms and then intervene to alter the destructive cycle of avoidance-based coping that leads to an ever-widening pattern of functional impairment?

There is one simple diagnostic rule to follow, with respect to identifying victims of trauma and violence: *always* be on the lookout for it. Anytime a patient presents with insomnia, for example, always ask the patient whether nightmares, night terrors, or night sweats are present. When a patient complains of having difficulty going outside, or won't go to a grocery except late at night or accompanied by someone, always inquire whether this is due to feeling unsafe or anxious around strangers. If a patient complains of being tense, jumpy, and unable to relax, inquire about any recent or past trauma that might be contributing to chronic overarousal and hypervigilance.

Another rule of thumb is to screen for PTSD symptoms when you get suspicious about the real cause of complaints like headaches, belly pain, and stomach upset. Ask something like, "Have you ever had anything horrible happen to you in your life, such that you can't stop thinking about it or have memories or nightmares about it?" Asking in this general way takes the pressure off the patient to have to "confess" to the exact nature of the trauma so you can learn that something bad has happened. You don't need to require the patient to explain the trauma in detail, because this will scare off many patients due to the anxiety and fear that go along with recollecting the event. It is simply necessary to be aware that something awful happened and let the patient, to the extent that time allows, influence the level of self-disclosure.

Once the trauma is identified, the primary care provider needs to provide brief, effective interventions. A structured and graded approach involving exposure to past traumas may be helpful. Brief, ongoing visits with an emphasis on skill training improve outcomes, even with homeless patients with multiple traumas who are using drugs (Desai, Harpaz-Rotem, Najavits, & Rosenheck, 2008). Interestingly, as patients improved in the study by Rani Desai and colleagues, the avoidance and arousal symptoms of PTSD improved most. A variety of real behavior change techniques can help the patient with a trauma history learn to hold still rather than avoid difficult TEAMS, take an observer stance, and pursue more value-consistent action more consistently. Think of the patient with trauma as being similar to patients with chronic pain syndrome. The typical patient with a history of trauma uses a variety of strategies to numb out in order to avoid memories and possible triggers of memories that might come up in various life situations (such as medical clinics, social events, or even living in housing as opposed to on the streets). Patients often develop a narrative explaining what often leads to a cycle of retraumatization. For example, women who were sexually abused as children may have life stories with themes of being broken, unlovable, unattractive, and deserving of maltreatment that comes their way.

The four most important directions for applying real behavior change strategies to trauma are to help patients accept the presence of unpleasant TEAMS without running from them or avoiding life situations that could produce them; learn to get in the present moment rather than numbing out, being drawn into the past, or both; see their self-stories or personal narratives as self-limiting efforts the mind makes to "make sense" of something that basically is a random and senseless act of the universe; and choose and pursue more meaningful lives. As indicated in the chapter-introduction box, we demonstrate interview questions and the Core Process Assessment Tool (CPAT), and then focus treatment on three processes, allowing us to apply five techniques. Remember that most often, your use of real behavior change interventions will involve fewer techniques. As teachers, we apply more, in order to give you more ideas.

Trauma Interventions	
<u>Love, Work, Play, and Health Questions</u>	
<u>Three-T and Workability Questions</u>	
<u>Core Process Assessment Tool (CPAT)</u>	
<u>Real Behavior Change Pocket Guide</u>	
Process	**Technique**
Experience the Present Moment	Balloon Breath
Use Observer Self to See Limiting Self-Stories	■ Be a Witness ■ <u>What Are Your Self-Stories?</u>
Strengthen Connection with Values and Sustain Value-Consistent Action	■ You Are Not Responsible; You Are Response Able ■ <u>Bull's-Eye Worksheet</u>

Remember, when this symbol appears next to discussions about a diagram or worksheet, you can find a copy online at <u>http://www</u> <u>.newharbingeronline.com/real-behavior-change-in-primary-care.html</u>.

CASE EXAMPLE: MARIA AND DR. MEYER

Maria, a twenty-six-year-old Cuban American female, sees Dr. Meyer for the first time for an urgent same-day visit she has requested.

Reason for Visit. Maria is requesting help with abdominal pain, insomnia, chronic headaches, nightmares, and stress at home.

Medical Status. Maria is otherwise healthy and has two children. Her blood pressure and pulse rate are quite elevated today, and she is visibly upset and tearful. She engages in continuous hand-wringing and leg bouncing. Her abdominal exam reveals no tenderness or other findings of concern.

Patient Concern. Maria is interested in getting help for her headaches, which have occurred on a daily basis for the last several months. She has a dull ache "on the left side that seems to get worse as the day goes on." She states that she sleeps about four to five hours a night because she can't relax. She reports that she is near the "breaking point" because she can't sleep—she has "terrible nightmares" and needs some medicine to help her deal with her stress.

Patient's Life Context. Maria separated from her husband of five years last week after he pushed her out of a moving vehicle during a marital argument. She reports that he has assaulted her both physically and sexually in the past; she called the police during one such argument and is currently working with them. She works full-time at a desk job and is now trying out the role of single parent. She stopped exercising on a regular basis about six months ago, when her husband accused her of having "eyes" for another man at her fitness club. She has gained fifteen to twenty pounds since then, because she tends to overeat when under stress. She doesn't abuse alcohol or drugs. She notes that she has bad dreams about "terrible things" that were done to her in the past.

Behavior-Change Interview

Because Maria is new to her practice, Dr. Meyer decides to use the Love, Work, Play, and Health Questions and the Three-T and Workability Questions to better understand Maria's chief complaints and how they impact her life context.

THE LOVE, WORK, PLAY, AND HEALTH QUESTIONS

Since Maria is obviously upset, Dr. Meyer's first objective is to develop rapport with her by asking about her life context. Sample worksheet 9.1 summarizes Maria's responses to the Love, Work, Play, and Health Questions.

SAMPLE WORKSHEET 9.1
Maria's Responses to the Love, Work, Play, and Health Questions

Question Area	Patient Responses
Love	Separated from husband, who abused her five times in the past year. Has two children at home (aged eight and five). She is afraid for her safety and feels her husband will come after her, but she is working with the police, who assure her they are watching and will respond promptly to any request. Her boyfriend as a teenager and the father of her oldest child were also abusive; "I just make lousy choices."
Work	Works full-time as a bilingual law clerk. Really likes her job and coworkers. Missed four days of work last month due to headaches.
Play	Likes to go to church (but not going now) and to the park with her children. Goes to eight-year-old's sports activities. At home, finds a warm bath sometimes helps with headaches; also likes to dance. Used to have several friends, but they were put off by her husband's rude behavior ("mostly when he drinks"); Maria avoids seeing them, because she thinks they'll criticize her for picking him over them.

Health	Doesn't use alcohol, drugs, or tobacco: "Never will; my dad was a drinker and a smoker. I got enough of that." No current exercise, did in past. Overeats when stressed. Slow to fall asleep and having "more and more nightmares." Daily headaches (8 on a scale of 1 to 10); acknowledges these are probably "stress" related.

Dr. Meyer now has a picture of Maria's strengths and a better context for understanding her recent marital separation. She admires Maria's concern for her children, her efforts to keep them away from the marital conflict, and her courage to work with the police. She suspects that Maria's recent trauma is triggering the reexperiencing of previous traumas.

THE THREE-T AND WORKABILITY QUESTIONS

Dr. Meyer now shifts to exploring Maria's current complaints, using the Three-T and Workability questions.

SAMPLE WORKSHEET 9.2
Maria's Responses to the Three-T and Workability Questions

Area	Questions	Patient Responses
Time	When did you first start to have trouble with nightmares? When did headaches start? More recently, any increase in problems? How often?	Seven years ago, after previous boyfriend held a knife to her throat and then beat her and threatened to kill her if she told anyone. About the same time. Yes, nightmares and headaches have worsened in past week. Nightmares most nights; headaches all day long.

Triggers	Did something trigger its worsening?	Husband got mad and pushed her out of the car at a red light on the way home from a restaurant. "We'd gone out for a romantic dinner, and he drank too much."
	What types of situations, events, or interactions make it worse?	Thinking about him makes everything worse.
	Better?	Staying home and cleaning helps. Being at work helps too. Told husband on the phone she was done and that the police would pick him up if he came to the house, but worries he will come anyway.
	Are there things inside of you that trigger this problem?	Memories of other times he hurt her—and her first partner too. Being alone in the bedroom, so sleeps on the couch.
	How do others react to your problem? What do they tell you to do?	Kids say they miss their dad. Peers at work are "covering" for her. File a restraining order (and she has); tell her she is a good person and deserves a good man.
Trajectory	Since the nightmares and headaches started, have they gotten worse or better, or stayed about the same?	Nightmares: sometimes more and sometimes less—more now. Headaches: wax and wane, tend to come in bunches—more now.

Workability Questions	What have you tried to cope with the sleep problems and headaches? How have these strategies worked over time? Are you getting the kind of results you want? When you use these strategies, are you getting some accidental negative results in other areas?	Get out of bed, have tea, try to wake up all the way, then go back to sleep. Try to "relax," take warm baths for headaches. "This works, but I don't get enough rest, and I'm tense and tired when I wake up. I know my worries and fears cause my headaches, but I don't know what to do." Staying home triggers overeating (and weight gain and feeling ugly); children also unhappy if she doesn't go out with them.

DR. MEYER: Maria, I am so sorry that you have been treated badly and harmed by someone you love. This is one of the worst things that can happen to us. It took a lot of courage to leave your husband and involve law officers. The headaches and nightmares are probably a part of this courageous and stressful change you are making. I want you to come back to see me next week; I have some ideas about new skills that might help you create a better life for yourself and your children. For now, I hope you will continue with the things that help: going to work, being with your children, and, oh yes, those warm baths. Oh, and I want you to think about the possibility of restarting some type of exercise.

Dr. Meyer ends the visit by reframing Maria's physical and emotional struggles. She explains that events such as a marital separation often trigger memories of other rough times and that taken together, the mental and physical systems get overloaded and cause problems with sleep and, often, headaches. Dr. Meyer compliments Maria on her devotion to her children and her persistence in continuing with her job. She also explains that the mind is sometimes helpful and sometimes less so. She gives examples of how Maria's mind helps her (such as suggesting that she exercise or play with her children) and examples of how it seems to be giving her unhelpful directions as well (such as *stay at home, don't try to see your friends*). Maria responds well to these ideas, stating that while this is a new way of thinking about her problems, it offers her some relief, "a different perspective."

Planning and Providing Treatment

After the first visit, Dr. Meyer takes a few moments to complete the CPAT to help guide her treatment planning, the results of which are in sample worksheet 9.3. Dr. Meyer concludes that, of the six core processes of psychological flexibility, those most likely to be pertinent to Maria's creating a better life are learning to experience the present moment when painful TEAMS appear, to use a bigger sense of self to see her self-story as a story rather than a fact, and to sustain the valued directions she is pursuing.

SAMPLE WORKSHEET 9.3 Maria's Core Process Assessment Tool (CPAT)

Six Core Processes: Psychological Rigidity	Patient Rating Today	Six Core Processes: Psychological Flexibility
Lives in the past or future	__X_____	Experiences the present moment
Disconnected from values	_____X_____	Strongly connected with values
Engages in impulsive, self-defeating action or inaction	_____X_____	Sustains value-consistent action
Stuck in limiting self-stories	_____X_____	Uses observer self to see limiting self-stories
Stuck in TEAMS and unworkable rules	_____X__	Steps back from TEAMS and unworkable rules
Actively avoids TEAMS	_____X__	Accepts TEAMS and focuses on action

Providing Follow-Up Care for Maria

When Maria comes for care a week later, she reports that she has been listening to her mind when it tells her to do healthy things. She and a friend from work have started going for walks at lunch. They don't talk about her problems much; they simply walk and chat about everyday things. Her headaches are less of a concern in the afternoons at work, and she is sleeping a little better.

EXPERIENCE THE PRESENT MOMENT

Dr. Meyer decides to pursue an intervention that will help Maria contact the present moment. She understands that trauma survivors tend to experience "lumpy" TEAMS. This means that all of these private experiences present themselves in a jumbled mass that's, on the one hand, very intrusive and overwhelming and, on the other hand, difficult to pull apart and experience individually. She wants to teach Maria how to hold still in the presence of lumpy TEAMS, stay focused in the moment, and not "blink and run" from them.

Balloon Breath. The following interaction describes Dr. Meyer's introduction of this exercise to Maria and Maria's response.

DR. MEYER: Maria, let's talk about your plans to resolve your relationship with your husband for the next five minutes, and I want you to watch what your mind does.

MARIA: [Nods affirmatively and immediately looks distressed.]

DR. MEYER: Is your mind presenting a lot of thoughts and feelings— memories and other things—right now?

MARIA: [Nods again.]

DR. MEYER: I want to help you find a place where you can just let this stuff be there, and stay in your skin at the same time. I want you to take several slow, deep breaths, thinking of your belly as a balloon. To empty the balloon, you tighten your abdomen and empty the balloon. Try taking four seconds to empty and then hold for one second; then take four seconds

165

to fill the balloon, hold a second; and repeat the cycle. If
you like, watch me for a few breaths, so you understand
what I'm asking you to do. [Dr. Meyer demonstrates, and
Maria imitates correctly.] Now, I want you to do this type
of breathing for a couple of minutes, just focusing on being
right here, right now. If you like, try saying "here" when you
empty the balloon and "now" when you fill it. When things
show up in your mind that distract you, gently bring your
attention back to here-and-now breathing.

Dr. Meyer and Maria talk about her pursuing a divorce for several
minutes, and Dr. Meyer supports her staying in the present moment (remember "here" and "now") when she appears to space out.

USE OBSERVER SELF TO SEE LIMITING
SELF-STORIES

Dr. Meyer sees an opportunity to build on the Balloon Breath and introduces the Be a Witness technique.

Be a Witness. Dr. Meyer asks Maria to continue to be present and, at the
same time, to witness or watch the appearance and passing of uncomfortable
thoughts, feelings, memories, and sensations. She guides Maria to continue
to direct her attention to the decision to end her marriage and then asks,
"What are you noticing?"

MARIA: My mind says I've failed, that it's my fault, that I didn't try
hard enough. If I could have been more reassuring to him,
he wouldn't have always been blowing up and scaring me and
the kids. Now my kids have to grow up without a father,
and it's my fault. But then, my mind is also saying that it's
not good for the kids to see him throwing things at home
and calling me names.

DR. MEYER: Okay, I want you to try saying to yourself, "I am a witness
for my thoughts, and I am having the thought called"—
whatever, maybe the "it's my fault" thought. When we are
able to notice sticky thoughts and feelings like this, we can

stay in the present. It's a special part of the self that does the witnessing; let's call this part the "observer self," okay?

MARIA: [Nods.]

DR. MEYER: Are any memories showing up?

MARIA: I remember falling on the pavement when Josh pushed me out of the car last week; he was already starting to take off at the red light, so I skinned my arm and bruised my hip and shoulder. It hurt a lot; I was really afraid. Now, I'm thinking about other times I've been scared I was going to be hurt. I want to stop, okay?

DR. MEYER: Let's go back to Balloon Breath: empty—one, two, three, four; hold for one second—and fill—one, two, three, four; hold for one second—and... [after a few breaths] to here and now. It's possible to be here and now, just watching thoughts, memories, and feelings called "scared" come and go; we don't need to avoid them or push them away. We can just use the observer self. Are you with me?

MARIA: Yes, I'm getting it; the breathing helps me calm down when I have the feeling called "scared."

DR. MEYER: Look around to see if you see any other feelings; sometimes fear will bring along some buddies.

MARIA: Guilt and shame about all of my bad choices. I've really messed up.

DR. MEYER: Okay, so guilt and shame show up, and the thought that sneaked in the door with them is that you messed up. Can you stay right here, right now, inside your skin while fear, guilt, shame, and self-blaming thoughts are in your mind?

MARIA: I'm trying. This is new for me.

While helping Maria enhance her ability to be present and witness painful TEAMS, Dr. Meyer models a neutral "simple awareness." With practice, Maria will develop her own simple awareness and learn to more easily separate from her stories about failing in relationships with men and being to blame. When we, as providers, treat patients who have had more than one abusive relationship, our minds may tell us, "She should have known better." At one level of analysis, it's easy to fall into blaming the victim for becoming a victim again. At the level of self-story, we can understand this pattern differently. Women who have been abused subsequently look for the "perfect" man who will treat them like a princess and promise never to do anything like the last guy did. When the romance phase ends and the abuse begins, the woman's self-story—*I've messed up* again—is confirmed. Here's a good rule of thumb: when the primary objective is to be safe in a relationship, the more unsafe the relationship may be.

What Are Your Self-Stories? Dr. Meyer wants to bring Maria's self-story into the visit to help her see this symbolic product in the same way she is beginning to witness her TEAMS. If she can see her self-story as a story, then she might be less dominated by its messages.

DR. MEYER: Maria, I noticed that something else has been showing up in the room along with your basic thoughts, memories, and emotions. It's a story you carry around about who you are; stories like that can influence where we are going. Can you bring more of that story into your mind, so we can use the observer self to see it as a story, rather than the truth, about you? Let's see, I think I heard *I always mess up, I don't try hard enough,* and *Because I mess up, my children have to suffer.* Am I hearing the story right?

MARIA: Yes, I think so; my father was very harsh with me. I was the oldest girl. He used to spank me with a belt—really for almost anything—and say he had to teach me a lesson. He always said I never tried hard enough and never learned, that I was a big disappointment.

DR. MEYER: Okay, so what does the story say about your future?

MARIA: That I will continue to mess up and be a disappointment to people I care about. Hmm, I think it even says I might as well go back with my husband, 'cause I won't find anyone better.

DR. MEYER: Okay, so this story says it knows what's going to happen in
               your life, say, in a year, two years, five years. Am I hearing
               that correctly?

MARIA: *(laughing slightly)* Yeah, I guess that seems a little crazy, but
               it sort of feels that way.

DR. MEYER: Well, you're not crazy for having a story; we all carry them
               around. I have mine; that's for sure. That's what minds do,
               and I suppose we have to take the bad with the good. The
               thing that has me scratching my head is how confidently
               your mind predicts what's going to happen to you over the
               years. I suppose, if you took your story literally, it would
               make life a pretty painful exercise. After all, the outcome is
               already decided: you don't get to live a vital, fulfilling life, at
               least according to your mind.

MARIA: I get very sad and depressed when I think about my future,
               my story.

DR. MEYER: Maria, there's a difference between being the storyteller and
               being the listener. I want you to practice being the listener:
               when you don't like the story your mind is giving you, you
               don't have to be bound by it. You can actually say "hello,
               story" and, in the world outside your mind, do things that
               contradict the story, like go to church, meet new people, and
               continue with your move to end a relationship that's been
               harmful to you.

SUSTAIN VALUE-CONSISTENT ACTION

Maria, like many survivors of violent trauma, is trying to "make sense"
of this horrific reality, and her story suggests that she "take the blame" for
the event. She is "to blame" for picking the wrong men, so in a weird way,
she "deserves" to be abused and traumatized. Her damaged sense of self will
make her vulnerable to further exploitative and predatory relationships, like
the one she is trying to leave.

You Are Not Responsible; You Are Response Able. Dr. Meyer wants to get Maria to look forward, not backward; she wants to help her develop a sense of "agency" that can propel her toward a healthy, loving relationship. Dr. Meyer introduces this technique as a foundation for bull's-eye behavior-change planning. This technique helps the patient shift from self-blame to more intentional choices.

DR. MEYER: Maria, it sounds as if blaming yourself is a big part of your story. If you are to blame for being involved with men who mistreat you, then it might mean that you deserve bad things that happen to you; is that right?

MARIA: I guess I do sort of think I have to settle for who's interested in me or I'll just be alone. That's what my husband said: "You can't leave me 'cause no one else would want you."

DR. MEYER: So, Maria, your story tells you that if you are responsible, you are to blame and you deserve to suffer. I think you are responsible but in a different way. You are response *able* [Dr. Meyers writes "response <u>able</u>"], meaning you are alive and able to choose your actions *now* and *in the future*. You are at a fork in the road: you can choose to go in the direction of responsibility, blame, and self-criticism, or you can go in the direction of your values about how you want to treat yourself and how you want to be treated by others. One road winds backward toward your past; the other goes forward to your future. Which road would give you the best chance of living the life you want to live?

MARIA: Well, I want to have a good life, and be respected and loved by others, so I guess I want to go on the road forward, the response *able* road.

Bull's-Eye Worksheet. Dr. Meyer uses the Bull's-Eye Worksheet to help Maria articulate her values regarding loving relationships, assess value–behavior discrepancy, and identify action steps. Sample worksheet 9.4 summarizes the results.

SAMPLE WORKSHEET 9.4
MARIA'S BULL'S-EYE WORKSHEET

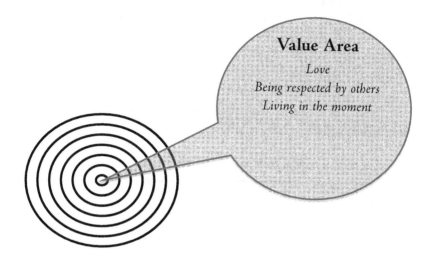

Value Area

Love
Being respected by others
Living in the moment

Action Step(s) (Short-Term):

1. *Get involved in church charity group.*

2. *Call up old friend and invite her to have a cup of coffee.*

3. *Practice Balloon Breath three times daily.*

4. *Join the women's health club for a month and go three to four times a week.*

5. *Use the observer self and be "response able."*

Maria returns in three weeks for a check on her headaches and behavior-change efforts. She reports that she has fewer and less-intense headaches, her stomachaches have stopped, and her bruising has resolved. She has practiced Balloon Breath every day, often many times throughout the day. She has met with an attorney and is proceeding with a divorce. She continues to walk at lunch with her work friend, and she has contacted a friend in the community, who told her, "You deserve someone who will love you and treat you with respect." She also joined the church charity group, and she and her children worked in a food drive the week before. Maria describes this experience as a chance to be around people who respect each other. At some point, she plans to join the church choir, but it seems like too big of a time commitment at this point. Maria has decided against the health club, for financial reasons. Dr. Meyer is delighted by Maria's behavior changes and tells her she is very "response *able*." She asks Maria to continue to practice the breathing and witnessing exercises: "These are new and important skills, and they will strengthen with practice."

SUMMARY

In this chapter, we have given you several powerful strategies for working with individuals suffering from trauma-related problems. Review the following points to check your mastery of key concepts:

- Trauma and the violence that often precedes it are far more prevalent than we often imagine, because trauma victims often do not reveal their "dark secret" but, rather, present with a variety of somatic complaints.

- The burden of humiliation, blame, and shame trauma victims carry with them can be lightened considerably when primary care providers take an open, accepting, and mindful stance and empower them to live in the moment and seize control of their life trajectory, one small step at a time.

- Techniques that enhance the present moment, such as Being a Witness, provide a sound foundation for building perspective-taking skills.

- When trauma victims can learn to ask *What are my self-stories?* and to understand that the self-stories are simply content in a larger context of self, they become empowered to move beyond the trap of a self-fulfilling prophecy.

- As the case example in this chapter illustrates, you don't have to do everything in one medical visit. Take your time, conduct a good ACT assessment, and then have the patient come back for an intervention planning session.

■ The concept of being response *able* helps trauma victims let go of guilt and shame and helps them make healthy choices that are consistent with their values.

■ When trauma victims begin to establish a more meaningful life, various aches and pains diminish, and we often see them less in the clinic and more in our communities, where they often play a special role in supporting others.

PREVIEW

In the next chapter, we will examine signs of burnout. Working in a primary care setting is a heroic endeavor and, like most heroic endeavors, is replete with risk.

PART 3

Applying Real Behavior Change Tools in Daily Practice

In this last part of the book, we invite you to shift your focus—and your new behavior-change tool kit—to yourself. Pursuing a meaningful medical career is challenging; plan for resilience! We provide you with tools to assess your risk of burnout and to build and rebuild a sustainable approach to your work—and your life.

CHAPTER 10

Better and Faster: The Risk of Burnout

To keep a lamp burning, we have to keep putting oil in it.

—Mother Teresa of Calcutta

The drive to provide care to more people, at a consistently high quality and a faster pace, adds exponentially to the already-high stress levels we experience in medical and nursing school, in residency training, and in daily practice. "More, better, and faster" is a philosophy that can reduce awareness, leading us into a process of giving more and more and receiving less and less. All too often, the twinkle dulls in the eye of a medical student whose passion was medicine, and the person has trouble reconnecting with the oil that fed the flame. This is the insidious process of burnout that's blazing through medical practice and training.

Indeed, prevalence estimates of burnout in primary care providers range from 26 percent to 65 percent (Linzer et al., 2009; Ratanawongsa et al., 2008). A recent study of European family doctors suggested that up to 43 percent experience *high* levels of burnout (European General Practice Research Network Burnout Study Group, 2008). Among medical students, the rate of burnout is 45 percent (Dyrbye et al., 2006). Estimates of burnout among medical residents range from 10 to 74 percent (Martini, Arfken, & Balon, 2006; Fahrenkopf et al., 2008), and in a study of pediatric residents, 20 percent screened positive for depression (Fahrenkopf et al., 2008). Depression is common among medical students (at 56 percent), and almost a quarter report at-risk use of alcohol (Dyrbye et al., 2006). Burnout among students and providers has a potentially huge impact on the availability of health care services today and in the future, as fewer physicians choose careers in primary care medicine, and many of those currently practicing contemplate a job change from medicine or early retirement.

In this chapter we will define burnout, and we will look at some of the factors and potential consequences associated with burnout in medical providers and trainees. We will also describe ways of assessing burnout and psychological flexibility in ourselves as health care providers and use the case of an attending physician, Dr. Jessica, to demonstrate self-assessment strategies. In chapter 12, we will use the case of Dr. Jessica to demonstrate use of intentional, specific coping strategies for improving resiliency in the face of burnout and for enhancing the experience of vitality in medical practice.

> Remember, when this symbol appears next to discussions about a diagram or worksheet, you can find a copy online at http://www .newharbingeronline.com/real-behavior-change-in-primary-care.html.

BURNOUT DEFINED

Burnout is the experience of long-term exhaustion and dwindling interest in normally meaningful work activities. While some theorists suggest that burnout is a personal and private problem, we believe a more productive perspective is to see it as a person-to-work interaction problem. This perspective allows us to look at burnout as a dynamic process, where separation of the individual from the surrounding context is artificial. This process-oriented view supports risk identification and development of meaningful interventions at the individual level as well as at the system-of-care level.

Christina Maslach and colleagues (2001) describe three main components of burnout: emotional exhaustion, depersonalization, and a lack of personal accomplishment. Emotional exhaustion is feeling emotionally drained and depleted as a result of excessive psychological demands, while depersonalization involves emotional distancing and feeling less connected to our patients. When our sense of personal accomplishment weakens, we may begin to feel less competent in our work. The Maslach Burnout Inventory (MBI) is a validated, self-administered survey that measures burnout in all three areas (Maslach, Jackson, & Leiter, 1996; Rafferty, Lemkau, Purdy, & Rudisill, 1986). It has been used in many studies, including studies involving primary care providers and trainees (Lieter & Maslach, 2009). We recommend using this tool if you suspect you have significant symptoms of burnout.

RISK FACTORS FOR BURNOUT

Medical students, residents, and practicing providers experience many of the circumstances that increase vulnerability to burnout. These factors occur in most practice and training environments, including the following four conditions (Linzer et al., 2009; Linzer et al., 2002; Deckard, Meterko, & Field, 1994).

- A weakening in sense of control in the work setting (for example, time pressure, panel size, paperwork, work hours, chaotic environments)

- An increase in responsibility for providing care to highly complex patients, in combination with a constriction of resources to support primary care management

- Limited availability of support from colleagues and spouse or partner (with colleagues making more demands and significant other offering less support to career)

- Practice in an organization that shifts toward a toxic work culture (for example, decreased quality emphasis, decreased trust in organization, decreased cohesiveness, and lack of alignment around values)

Students engaged in training for a health care profession experience additional risk factors. The typical trainee leaves his social support system, moves to a new community, and starts a new job—all at the same time. Intimate relationships tend to solidify or end at this juncture, and those who remain in committed relationships often struggle with prolonged periods of separation. The incidence of burnout increases as students proceed through medical school, and students most at risk for burnout are those who experience negative life events along with high professional demands (Dyrbye et al., 2006). While medical students and residents accept that their lives will be *temporarily* "imbalanced" during training (Ratanawongsa, Wright, & Carrese, 2007), the groundwork for living an imbalanced life is often established during this period and is carried forward into practice. In other words, living an imbalanced life for any extended period of time allows unhealthy lifestyle habits to form that can later put the individual at risk.

CONSEQUENCES: THE STING OF BURNOUT

Burnout has significant consequences for trainees, practitioners, their families, and their patients. Burnout promotes use of behavioral avoidance strategies (such as participating less often in activities with friends and family, use of alcohol as a calming strategy at the end of the day), which then result in a lowered quality of life. Practitioners with higher levels of burnout appear to use more sick leave and report greater use of tobacco, alcohol, and psychotropic medication (European General Practice Research Network Burnout Study Group, 2008). A study of internal medicine residents showed high burnout scores to be associated with self-perceived errors (West, Tan, Habermann, Sloan, & Shanafelt, 2009). In another study, researchers reviewed the charts of pediatric residents, trying to find an association between burnout and medical errors. Interestingly, while burnout was not associated with documented medical errors, it correlated with depression levels in the residents (Fahrenkopf et al., 2008). In a study of physician–patient interaction, physician burnout did not result in decreased ratings of patient-centeredness, patient satisfaction, confidence, trust, quality of care, or increased errors. However, patients of high-burnout physicians used more negative statements, such as criticism, and disagreed more with their providers or other people in the clinic outside the encounter (Ratanawongsa et al., 2008; Linzer et al., 2009). High levels of burnout have also been associated with increased intent to leave one's current practice, and dissatisfied physicians are two to three times more likely to leave medicine (Landon, Reschovsky, Pham, & Blumenthal, 2006).

BURNOUT PREVENTION AND RECOVERY

While you may be unable to make immediate changes to your work environment, you can change how you respond to it, starting today. You can dampen the discomfort you experience from avoiding or suppressing your emotions, fusing with your thoughts about work and its meaning, and reacting impulsively to your staff or loved ones. You can fine-tune your lifestyle and make choices based on your values. The same ACT processes and interventions you are learning to use with your patients can work for you. For example, a study of Canadian family physicians reported that they benefited from applying ACT or real behavior change strategies, including acceptance of limitations, use of humor and spiritual strategies, prioritizing values, and applying self-reflection and self-awareness (Lee et al., 2009). A recent randomized, controlled trial of psychotherapists compared a group trained in ACT with a group undergoing multicultural competence training to assess changes in burnout and stigmatizing attitudes toward substance-addicted patients. Results suggested that the ACT-trained group had greater improvement on self-report measures of burnout and significantly decreased stigmatizing attitudes toward patients (Hayes, Bissett, et al., 2004). By combining practices of acceptance and mindfulness with commitment to behaviors that are consistent with the core values of pursuing a medical career, you can strengthen your ability to respond to the daily challenges of patient care with thoughtfulness and positive energy.

There is compelling evidence that you can reduce or prevent burnout, but first you must gain a better understanding of what factors might be increasing your risk. As you can see in the chapter-introduction box, we introduce four tools (two new and two demonstrated in earlier clinical chapters) for assessing sources of personal and professional stress and identifying protective factors that may enhance your resiliency. We recommend printing a copy of the PCP-AAQ (appendix B) and the PCP-SC (appendix C) from the website (or copying them from the appendixes) before reading further.

Provider Burnout Assessment Tools

Primary Care Provider Acceptance and Action Questionnaire (PCP-AAQ)

Primary Care Provider Stress Checklist (PCP-SC)

Love, Work, Play, and Health Questions

Three-T and Workability Questions

ASSESSING BURNOUT RISK AND PROTECTIVE FACTORS IN YOUR LIFE

A recent study of intensive care nurses reported a positive correlation between scores on a general measure of emotional avoidance (the Acceptance and Action Questionnaire, described later) and measures of depersonalization and emotional exhaustion scores on the Maslach Burnout Inventory (Losa Iglesias et al., 2010). To help you evaluate your underlying vulnerability, we provide a version of the Acceptance and Action Questionnaire (AAQ-II) designed specifically for medical providers. Your score on the Primary Care Provider Acceptance and Action Questionnaire (PCP-AAQ) will help you get an estimate of your *current* level of psychological flexibility. Greater psychological flexibility will improve your resiliency in the face of the ongoing stresses associated with providing medical services, and using real behavior change strategies will help you use more flexibility-promoting strategies inside and outside of the clinic. A second tool, the Primary Care Provider Stress Checklist (PCP-SC), will help you identify specific sources of stress. Both the PCP-AAQ and the PCP-SC offer "snapshot" information, so repeated use can help you stay in touch with yourself and make changes strategically.

Primary Care Provider Acceptance and Action Questionnaire (PCP-AAQ)

The Primary Care Provider Acceptance and Action Questionnaire (PCP-AAQ) is a way to take stock of subtle processes that impact your resilience. The PCP-AAQ (appendix B) is based on an empirically validated measure of experiential avoidance (see the website or appendix A for a copy of the Acceptance and Action Questionnaire [AAQ-II], Hayes, Strosahl, et al., 2004). The PCP-AAQ offers an estimate of your current ability to use acceptance strategies during emotionally challenging moments in practice— while pursuing personally meaningful action. Print the PCP-AAQ from the website (or copy appendix B) and complete the form. It usually takes five to ten minutes. Higher scores suggest greater flexibility, which often means more resilience in the face of burnout. If your score is low, you stand to benefit from the resiliency-building techniques described in the next chapter.

Primary Care Provider Stress Checklist (PCP-SC)

The Primary Care Provider Stress Checklist (PCP-SC) provides information about specific sources of stress in the work setting. A copy of the PCP-SC is available online and in appendix C. We suggest printing it and responding to it now. Then, you'll have the information you need to make a plan. To complete the PCP-SC, use a scale from 0 (not stressful) to 6 (extremely stressful) to rate the level of stress you typically experience in thirty-seven different circumstances. The items cover six general areas:

- Interactions with patients

- Practice management

- Administrative issues

- Education and learning requirements

- Relationships with colleagues

- Balance between work and "the rest of life"

As for scoring on the PCP-SC, you sum your scores in each of the six areas. Then, you transfer your scores to a summary table and divide by the

183

number indicated in the "divide by" column. For each area, you will have a stress score ranging between 0 and 1. Think of these scores as percentages. A score of 1 in the Interactions with Patients area suggests you are experiencing a maximum amount of stress (100 percent) when interacting with patients, which might mean that most of your patients are highly complex, at-risk patients. A score of .17, or 17 percent, in Relationships with Colleagues might suggest that you have strong support from colleagues and that this area may enhance your resilience in practicing medicine. You can obtain your Total PCP-SC Score by dividing the sum of the scores of all six Category Totals by 222 (alternatively, add all six Stress Scores and divide by 6). This total provides an indication of your overall stress level, while the area scores provide more-specific information you can use to formulate a coping plan.

Identifying the source of your stress is a critical step in developing an intentional, active coping plan. Problem-focused coping can help you address specific sources of stress. Problem-focused strategies involve advocating for external, organizational change; applying new personal and spiritual strategies to alleviate stresses you experience in the workplace; or both.

CASE EXAMPLE: DR. JESSICA

Dr. Jessica, a fifty-year-old senior family physician, feels "burned out." She's been working in her current practice, providing full-spectrum family medicine, for fifteen years. While she continues to love family medicine, she says she is "tired of the long hours, overwhelming paperwork, demanding patients, and not seeing my family enough." The hospital report on "Best Practices" noted that Dr. Jessica recently failed to document echo results on a couple of patients she admitted for congestive heart failure. The report also noted that she's behind on her office dictations. She had a few complicated pregnant patients earlier this year. One patient went into labor and delivery with a prolapsed cord and required a stat C-section. Another patient had a fetal death in utero (FDIU) at thirty-six weeks gestation. No etiology for the death was identified on autopsy. Both patients still respect Dr. Jessica and want her to continue to be their doctor, but she has bad dreams about the deliveries and feels guilty at times—worrying that she should have picked up something in the prenatal period about the FDIU incident.

She feels as if her kids (a twelve-year-old boy and a fourteen-year-old girl) are growing up and, she says, "I haven't spent enough time with them."

She hasn't been able to attend many of their soccer games and school plays. She's thankful that her husband's parents live locally, help out with the kids, and go to their performances. She doesn't see much of her husband, Bob, and while she feels confident about their relationship, she worries about the "distance growing between us." Bob is an engineering consultant and is able to stay home and work, but he now wants to take on new assignments that require him to work in the office and to travel out of state occasionally.

Dr. Jessica has a hard time relaxing after work, so she drinks one to two glasses of wine. She used to ride a bicycle on a regular basis but stopped doing that about six months ago, when one of her partners took a leave of absence and she picked up extra hours to provide coverage. Recently, her husband said he thought she was depressed: "Even when you're at the house, you're not really with us." While her husband understands how demanding her work is, he misses her and wants "the old" her back. She feels she has no energy to attend to the kids or to him, but she tries to anyway. She doesn't seem to enjoy her work, and she feels sad because it used to give her a strong sense of accomplishment. She's concerned that one glass of wine is turning into two and sometimes three. She has decided, "It's time to either make some personal changes or seek professional help." She values being "a lifelong learner" and believes that some of the real behavior change techniques might help her. First, she decides to start by completing the PCP-AAQ and the PCP-SC.

Dr. Jessica's PCP-AAQ Results

Dr. Jessica's PCP-AAQ total score is 58 (total scores range from 0 to 120, with higher scores indicating greater psychological flexibility). These results suggest to Dr. Jessica that she can enhance her resiliency to the ongoing stress of medical practice by learning skills designed to promote greater psychological flexibility. In particular, she notes that she has a hard time accepting her memories of the FDIU incident and is also critical of herself in other domains of life.

Dr. Jessica's PCP-SC Results

Dr. Jessica's PCP-SC results deliver a powerful message to her (see sample worksheet 10.1). First, she feels validated: she isn't "losing it" as much as she is under a lot of pressure, and her daily struggle with administrative issues and the long-lost balance between work and play are heavy hitters in her experience of burnout.

SAMPLE WORKSHEET 10.1
Dr. Jessica's PCP-SC Results

PCP-SC Source of Stress	Category Total	Divide By	Stress Score
Interactions with Patients	16	42	.38
Practice Management	17	36	.47
Administrative Issues	23	36	.64
Education/Learning	11	36	.31
Relationships with Colleagues	17	36	.47
Balance Between Work and the "Rest of Life"	26	36	.72
Total PCP-SC Score	110	222	.50

Dr. Jessica's Love, Work, Play, and Health Self-Assessment

In an effort to further her understanding of her present situation, Dr. Jessica answers the Love, Work, Play, and Health Questions in regard to herself (see sample worksheet 10.2).

SAMPLE WORKSHEET 10.2
Dr. Jessica's Responses to the Love, Work, Play, and Health Questions

Area	Responses
Love	Live with husband of fifteen years and our two healthy children. Relationship with husband is solid, but I feel I'm losing my connection with him and the kids. He's been the primary homemaker.
Work	Full-time in family practice doing full-spectrum care. Used to enjoy work, but now less tolerant of difficult patients, tired of the hours and paperwork. Less confident about obstetrics.
Play	Not much. Used to ride a bike regularly alone or with some girlfriends. Haven't seen my friends in months and haven't exercised in longer than that. Have a glass or two of wine at night.
Health	Worried, feel like I'm starting to depend on wine at night. No illegal or prescription drugs. My husband cooks pretty healthfully, but I have sweets at night if I have trouble sleeping. Recurrent bad dreams, mostly about babies, problems with delivery. Having lots of trouble falling asleep and staying asleep.

Dr. Jessica's Responses to the Three-T and Workability Questions

Dr. Jessica's responses to the Three-T and Workability Questions are summarized in sample worksheet 10.3.

SAMPLE WORKSHEET 10.3
Dr. Jessica's Responses to the Three-T and Workability Questions

Area	Questions	Responses
Time	Focused on sleep (her main concern)	Problems with sleep started in spring, about a year ago. Things got worse during the summer when my hours increased at work.
Triggers	What do you think is causing the problem? Did anyone or anything set it off?	I think about work a lot. I spend so much time there, and it's hard to leave work at work. I had some tough deliveries about a year ago. Started having bad dreams about them. Figured it would get better with time and started having a glass of wine to help me get to sleep. Then things got worse when one of my partners took a leave of absence. It meant more hours for me and less time at home.

Trajectory	What's this problem been like over time? Have there been times when it has been more of a concern? What have you tried in the past?	I think it's gotten worse because it's affecting my family. My kids don't ask me to go to their games anymore. I'm tired all the time, don't have the energy to do things with them, and use work as an excuse. I'm worried that I'm failing at work and at home.
Workability Questions	What have you tried to cope with this problem? How has it worked? What has been the cost of using these strategies in terms of your values?	I've been keeping my nose to the grindstone and trying to get my work done. The alcohol probably isn't helping in the long run. It used to help me get to sleep, but it's not even doing that anymore, and I feel bleary-eyed the next day.

Dr. Jessica summarizes the results from the Three-T and Workability Questions this way: "I've been having a hard time sleeping since the difficult deliveries occurred a while back, and it's worsened since I started covering for my partner. I spend less time with my family, and I feel guilty and less connected. Alcohol probably helps me numb myself to some of the feelings and thoughts twirling around in my head, but the price I'm paying in regard to my family, my friends, and my own health isn't worth it."

SUMMARY

In this chapter, you have learned about burnout and how insidious and pervasive it is. We have provided information to help you better understand the various risk factors for burnout in medical practice. No one is immune to these forces, so we recommend periodically checking in and assessing your level of burnout, as well as the factors that may either protect you from burnout or make you more vulnerable to it. In addition, we introduced two survey tools for you to use to assess your level of psychological flexibility (PCP-AAQ) and the stress you are experiencing in six areas of your medical practice (PCP-SC). Knowing what is stressing you out is the first step to taking meaningful action. Check your comprehension by reading through these additional summary points:

- Burnout involves emotional exhaustion, depersonalization, and lack of a sense of personal accomplishment.

- Patients treated by providers with more signs of burnout report more negative interactions with their PCPs and affiliated staff compared to patients treated by providers with low burnout levels.

- Burnout does not appear to be associated with increased risk of making a medical error.

- People training for or working in medical careers are often exposed to factors in the work environment that may trigger burnout (for example, time pressure, increased panel size, long work hours, reduction of management support services, and limited support from colleagues and primary partner).

- The PCP-AAQ is an instrument that will help you assess your current level of psychological flexibility and estimate your resiliency to burnout.

- The PCP-SC is an instrument that helps you identify specific sources of stress and gain an overall sense of your stress level.

- You can use the PCP-AAQ and the PCP-SC (along with the Love, Work, Play, and Health Questions and the Three-T and Workability Questions) to create an information base for developing a plan to enhance your resiliency.

PREVIEW

In this chapter, we've helped you assess whether you are susceptible to burnout by looking at your level of professional stress and your psychological flexibility in the face of stress. In the next chapter, we'll show you how to enhance your psychological flexibility and cope with the stresses of a career in medicine.

CHAPTER 11

Provider Wellness: Preventing Burnout and Improving Job Satisfaction

Learning is experience. Everything else is just information.

—Albert Einstein

The decision to enter into the field of family medicine carries with it the potential for both great joy and great sorrow. On the one hand, you are in a position to help your patients improve their health and well-being, sometimes in the face of long odds. At other times, however, there is an absence of joy, because long hours and occasional unfortunate outcomes create tension, self-doubt, and withdrawal (as in the case of Dr. Jessica in the previous chapter). These are the hard times of being a family practitioner; they are part of your "contract" in being a medical service provider. To know great joy, you must also be willing to know great sorrow. At times like this, it is easy to get discouraged or lose sight of your underlying values. If you can stay connected with the underlying purpose of your mission as a PCP, you can weather the storm.

This chapter will help you clarify your mission and incorporate strategies that promote psychological flexibility in your daily life at home and at work. We will continue the story of Dr. Jessica (from the previous chapter) and see how she pursues psychological resilience and makes some long overdue changes in her professional practice and personal life. As you can see in the chapter-introduction box, our case targets three processes and illustrates five techniques.

Provider Wellness Interventions

Process	Technique
Strengthen Connection with Values	Retirement Party/Tombstone Bull's-Eye Professional and Personal Values Assessment
Step Back from TEAMS and Unworkable Rules	Velcro Clouds in the Sky
Use Observer Self to See Limiting Self-Stories	Circles of Self Miracle Question
Sustain Value-Consistent Action	Burnout Prevention and Recovery Plan

Remember, when this symbol appears next to discussions about a diagram or worksheet, you can find a copy online at http://www .newharbingeronline.com/real-behavior-change-in-primary-care.html.

CASE EXAMPLE: DR. JESSICA

Based on the results of her self-assessments (see the previous chapter), Dr. Jessica thinks through her situation using the Core Process Assessment Tool (CPAT). She wants to identify the processes that could give her the "most bang for the buck" in terms of burnout recovery. She decides to work to strengthen her connection with values, reasoning that it is possible to balance pursuit of a nourishing personal life with a meaningful medical practice. She also sees a need to strengthen her skill in stepping back from TEAMS and unworkable rules, as well as accepting TEAMS while acting in ways that are consistent with her values. Using alcohol and "working harder" are probably behavioral avoidance strategies that don't work for her in the long run. She decides to try several of the techniques in the Real Behavior Change Pocket Guide.

Strengthen Connection with Values

Dr. Jessica's first step is to sit down and complete a value clarification exercise that will help her identify which values are important to her, and the degree to which she is following them.

Retirement Party/Tombstone. To better connect with her values, Dr. Jessica decides to complete the personal and professional values exercise, Retirement Party (appendix J). As you can see in sample worksheet 11.1, the instructions for this exercise ask that you imagine being at your own retirement party, where friends and colleagues remember you for what you contributed over the course of your career. This exercise tends to create a "big picture" awareness of where you are headed in your professional life and can, at times, be both troubling and helpful. Tombstone, another version of this exercise, involves inviting the professional (or a patient, for that matter) to think through what he would hope to see on his tombstone. While requiring only minutes to describe, it supports a strong connection with values.

SAMPLE WORKSHEET 11.1
Dr. Jessica's Responses to the Retirement Party Worksheet

Retirement Party Worksheet
Instructions: For each of the following four life areas, describe your core values. For example, if you were at your own retirement party, what would you like to hear other people say about what you stood for, the mark you left generally, what your behavior over the years demonstrated about your personal beliefs? **Studying or Practicing Medicine (for example, your efforts to learn or practice):** She was compassionate and could explain things to her patients in a way they could understand. She kept up to date on evidence-based medicine and applied it to her practice. She made sure things got done for her patients. The staff always enjoyed working with her because she treated everybody with respect and worked as a team member. **Professional Relationships:** She cherished her relationships with colleagues, nurses, and staff, and she was well liked by everyone. She was ever willing to cover for her colleagues and often sacrificed her personal time to do so. She enjoyed talking medicine with her colleagues and was always available for a curbside consultation, even if it interrupted her practice. She treated everyone as an equal. **Teaching Medicine (for example, your efforts to prepare others for medical careers):** She was an excellent teacher and mentor for medical students and residents who spent time with her. She was very patient, and she understood the difficulties of learning such a complex subject. She gained genuine pleasure from teaching medicine to others. **Balancing Professional and Private Lives:** Her family and friends always felt loved and appreciated by her. Even though she didn't get to lots of the children's games and other activities because of her busy schedule, they knew she always cared and that she tried to go. She always took time to ask them about their day and was interested in their friends and activities. Her husband admired the work she did with her patients and felt fortunate to be married to someone bright and caring. They went through some rough times together dealing with their careers and family but always seemed to work it out, and they knew deep down that their love and commitment would last a lifetime.

Bull's-Eye Professional and Personal Values Assessment. Jessica reads her responses several times and observes that her actions of late do not demonstrate some of her core values and ideals. She decides to further explore value–behavior discrepancies in her professional and personal lives by completing the Bull's-Eye Professional and Personal Values Assessment (appendix K). This exercise helps students and professionals better connect with their values, identify areas of discrepancy, and plan and pursue value-consistent actions over time. In this exercise, draw a star in each of the four quadrants—Practice of Medicine, Professional Relationships, Teaching Medicine, and Balance of Personal and Professional Lives—to indicate your value consistency over the past month (see sample worksheet 11.2 for Dr. Jessica's responses).

SAMPLE WORKSHEET 11.2
Dr. Jessica's Responses to the Bull's-Eye
Professional and Personal Values Assessment

Name: ___Dr. Jessica___   Date: ___June 11, 2010___

Bull's-Eye Professional and Personal Values Assessment

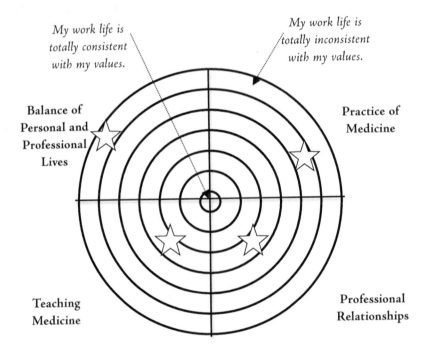

Instructions: Place an "X" or draw a star in each of the four quadrants to represent the degree to which you have been living according to your values in each area during the past month.

Dr. Jessica observes that her biggest value–behavior discrepancies are in balancing her professional and personal lives (sixth ring out from the center) and in her practice of medicine (fifth ring out from the center). She realizes she has lost sight of how to live by her values during day-to-day medical practice. She struggles with "difficult" patients, the same patients she once found complex and fascinating. She has started to distance herself emotionally from her patients, colleagues, and staff—even her family. She reasons that she is trying to conserve her energy, but she is only getting more tired. Obstetrical care once brought her a great deal of pleasure, a "payback" that counterbalanced the stress of a busy practice. While the balance of her personal and professional lives is lopsided toward work, she feels less of a sense of accomplishment and connection. Her choices to work extra hours, numb herself to her feelings, and reduce time with friends and family are draining her sense of vitality, purpose, and meaning. She decides to hang the Bull's-Eye Professional and Personal Values Assessment and Retirement Party worksheets on her refrigerator to remind herself and show her family that change is happening.

Step Back from TEAMS and Unworkable Rules

As she experiences a stronger connection with her values, Dr. Jessica decides it is time to shore up other psychological processes that could enhance her health and happiness. She decides to focus on acceptance and defusion skills (review chapter 3). "Stuffing" her thoughts and feelings isn't working, and she needs new ways of dealing with them. Defusion involves stepping back and learning to look *at* your thoughts rather than *from* your thoughts, to recognize that they are thoughts, not truths. While Dr. Jessica knows logically that there is nothing she could have done to prevent the FDIU and that her patient appreciated her compassionate presence at the time of the delivery and afterward, she continues to "get hooked" by these distressing TEAMS about the FDIU. She decides to try two techniques to improve her skills in this area: Velcro and Clouds in the Sky.

Velcro. This exercise involves identifying sticky TEAMS, ones that seem to have Velcro on them so that they attach immediately to invisible Velcro strips on our foreheads. Once they are attached, we can no longer see them as just thoughts or feelings. You write them on small sticky notes and stick them on your forehead, chest, and so on, where you can see them when you look in a mirror. As you look in the mirror, it helps to read them aloud. Dr. Jessica writes her TEAMS (see sample worksheet 11.3) one by one on bright-pink sticky notes and then places them on her forehead, chest, and shoulders. When she reads the "Memories" element, tears fill her eyes.

SAMPLE WORKSHEET 11.3
Dr. Jessica's Velcro Exercise

Thoughts	If I were a better doctor, I would have figured out what was going on before the FDIU happened. Can I keep doing this kind of work?
Emotions	Sadness, guilt, worry.
Associations	Every time I see a new OB patient, I think about the FDIU and whether it will happen again.
Memories	Seeing the mother sitting upright in bed with her husband's arm around her, holding the dead baby wrapped in a pink blanket. Both tearful, but looking at the baby lovingly.
Sensations	Pain in chest, pressure behind eyes, tightness in throat.

She looks in the mirror for a long time, repeating each TEAMS element aloud, then silently. She can't help but laugh at the sight of all the pink notes sticking to her and the tears running down her cheeks. She then proceeds to take one sticky note off at a time, read it aloud, and then place it on the inside cover of a journal she bought. (Years ago, she had a habit of writing in a diary, and it was helpful). These TEAMS will become a chapter in her new journal, one of many she will write in learning how to accept both the painful and precious moments in her life.

Step Back from TEAMS and Unworkable Rules

Dr. Jessica is painfully aware of how she struggles to avoid memories about the FDIU. They trouble her the most at night, and she often spends hours trying to think of other things just to keep the unwanted memories of the FDIU out of her mind. She is intrigued by the Clouds in the Sky intervention because, in their childhood, she and her older sister spent many an afternoon identifying animal shapes in the clouds.

Clouds in the Sky. This exercise involves identifying troubling TEAMS and just noticing them when they show up, without evaluating them or struggling to change them in any way. As a way of promoting this type of acceptance, you imagine resting beneath a shade tree on a warm day. You lie down on the grass, look up at the sky, and begin to watch the clouds. It's a day when the clouds are moving and reforming. The goal is to take each TEAMS element, place it on a cloud, and watch it with your mind's eye as it gently drifts around, merging and separating, and separating from and merging with the other clouds, finding its way to new and different shapes and eventually passing from view. Dr. Jessica thinks this technique might help her work with TEAMS about recent problems that tend to show up at night concerning pregnant patients. As a nightly practice, Dr. Jessica begins to invite distressing TEAMS and practices, placing them one by one on a cloud in the sky. She watches as the cloud forms and drifts by, and sometimes she cries. After working with this imagery for five minutes, she stretches and listens to a favorite piece of music before heading to bed. This proves helpful, so she decides to try it at work when troubling TEAMS show up, as they sometimes do before appointments with new pregnant patients. Dr. Jessica begins to notice a change in the way she experiences these unpleasant TEAMS. She is developing the ability to be aware and accepting of them without feeling compelled to do anything about their presence.

Sustain Value-Consistent Action

A life with vitality is filled with activities that contribute to your health and well-being and to that of your loved ones. Dr. Jessica is ready to develop and commit to an action plan.

Burnout Prevention and Recovery Plan. This exercise (appendix L) helps you develop a specific plan of action for promoting your health and well-being, given your ongoing experience of high levels of professional stress. To help you think broadly about techniques you might want to use, review the Real Behavior Change Pocket Guide (appendix H), looking closely at process areas where you feel you need to strengthen your skills. Choose techniques you believe you can incorporate into your daily life, and think through various action plans you want to pursue. Dr. Jessica's plan is in sample worksheet 11.4. She tapes a copy of it on the inside of her office door at work and her bedroom door at home. Her husband is pleased to see it, which leads to a good discussion between them. We recommend including your significant others (spouse, life partner, adult children, friends, siblings, and so on) in your plan to change your lifestyle habits. Not only can they hold you accountable and keep you on track, but they are also an important source of positive reinforcement—an important part of sustaining behavior change.

SAMPLE WORKSHEET 11.4
Dr. Jessica's Responses to the Burnout Prevention and Recovery Plan

Burnout Prevention and Recovery Plan

To help reduce your risk of burnout, describe specific behaviors you intend to use, when you will use them, and how often for each of the following four skill areas. Try to respond to at least two areas initially and add more plans later. The more specific your plan, the more likely you are to follow it!

Practice of Acceptance: *Defusion—Tonight and every night for the next week, start practicing the Clouds in the Sky exercise before bed and then again whenever TEAMS about the FDIU or other things going on at work come to my mind when I am in bed.*

Acceptance—*Write a chapter about the FDIU in my journal and then start figuring out "names of other chapters" I might write in my journal.*

Practice of Mindfulness (for example, present-moment awareness, contacting observer self): *Save for later!*

Practice of Contact with Personal Values: *I'll keep my bull's-eye posted on my refrigerator door. That way, when I get up every morning, I'll see it first thing, be reminded of what's truly important in my life, and avoid getting distracted from my goals. My family will also be able to see it, realize I'm committed to them, hold me accountable, and welcome me back into family life!*

Practice of Value-Consistent Daily Action: *I will set up a meeting this week with the practice manager and my partners, and let them know I can no longer continue to cover the extra night call and clinic sessions. I'll suggest we figure out a plan for the next six weeks that distributes the coverage among all of us and that we also consider some flextime during the day to compensate for the extra night sessions. That way I'll be less drained and more likely to catch some of the kids' school and sports activities. I'll ask Bob and the kids if they are willing to go for a bike ride or a walk with me at least once a week, and I'll ask Bob to go out on a "date" with me, without the kids, at least twice a month.*

After years of long hours, intimate contact with patient suffering, and unending demands from the health care bureaucracy, it's easy for your connection to core values to weaken. Dr. Jessica connects with her values, learns new techniques to deal with some painful experiences, reimagines her life, and uses the bull's eye and her family support to pursue greater vitality.

SUMMARY

While practice environments certainly differ in the amount of stress and burnout they generate, there are few contexts in medicine that are low stress. This means that you will most likely have to come to grips *repeatedly* with finding an optimal balance between your personal and professional lives. This will likely require learning new skills; let's review what this chapter offers you in this quest:

■ The Retirement Party technique is a powerful value clarification exercise for students, residents, and seasoned providers.

■ The Bull's-Eye Professional and Personal Values Assessment and the Burnout Prevention and Recovery Plan are useful tools for reflection. We recommend using them on an annual basis, perhaps at staff retreats.

■ We need a variety of tools to help us let go of the painful experiences we have in the practice of medicine. Remember the Velcro and Clouds in the Sky techniques; many students and providers find them useful.

■ During your busy days at the clinic, when you refer to the Real Behavior Change Pocket Guide (appendix H), think about yourself and your colleagues, as well as your patients. Learning is a lifelong endeavor!

APPENDIX A

Acceptance and Action Questionnaire (AAQ-II)

Following is a list of statements. Rate how true each statement is for you by circling a number next to it. Use the scale below to make your choice.

1	2	3	4	5	6	7
Never true	Very rarely true	Seldom true	Sometimes true	Often true	Almost always true	Always true

1. It's okay if I remember something unpleasant.   1 2 3 4 5 6 7

2. My painful experiences and memories make it difficult for me to live a life that I would value.   1 2 3 4 5 6 7

3. I'm afraid of my feelings.   1 2 3 4 5 6 7

4. I worry about being unable to control my worries and feelings.   1 2 3 4 5 6 7

5. My painful memories prevent me from having a fulfilling life.   1 2 3 4 5 6 7

6. I am in control of my life.   1 2 3 4 5 6 7

7. Emotions cause problems in my life.   1 2 3 4 5 6 7

8. It seems as if most people are handling their lives better than I am.   1 2 3 4 5 6 7

9. Worries get in the way of my success.   1 2 3 4 5 6 7

10. My thoughts and feelings do not get in the way of how I want to live my life.   1 2 3 4 5 6 7

Scoring Instructions: Reverse-score items 2, 3, 4, 5, 7, 8, and 9. Reversing a score means you take the number opposite of the number circled (for example, a circled score of 2 is scored as 6, a score of 3 as 5, and so on). After reverse-scoring items 2, 3, 4, 5, 7, 8, and 9, sum all scores to get the total score.

Interpreting Scores: Higher scores suggest greater psychological flexibility. The mean score for a university student and community sample was 50.72, while the mean for a sample of people seeking treatment for substance abuse was 39.80. Remember, your scores will change over time and you can use real behavior change strategies to raise your score.

(For more information, see Bond et al., 2010.)

Primary Care Provider Acceptance and Action Questionnaire (PCP-AAQ)

Name: _____ Date: _____

Rate the truth of each statement as it applies to your experience in providing medical care *at this moment*. Use the following scale from 0 to 6 and place a number in the box by each item.

0	1	2	3	4	5	6
Never true	Very rarely true	Seldom true	Sometimes true	Often true	Almost always true	Always true

	1. I am comfortable sitting quietly when my patient is crying.
	2. I accept that I cannot make my patients change unhealthy habits or manage their diseases better.
	3. I allow myself to experience anger, sadness, or frustration in my daily practice of medicine.
	4. I won't sacrifice my personal time to catch up on office work, even though it would help me feel less stressed at work.

	5. I'm able to empathize with my patients even when I'm running behind schedule.
	6. The pressure of daily practice doesn't prevent me from enjoying myself at work.
	7. Helping patients with emotional problems is a rewarding part of my medical practice, even though it can be emotionally draining at times.
	8. I am able to manage difficult interactions with staff or colleagues, even though my own thoughts or emotions may be negative.
	9. I don't take my work stress home with me.
	10. Accepting my negative reactions to a stressful situation is part of how I cope with it.
	11. I allow myself to feel guilty when I make a medical error.
	12. Despite the stress of daily practice, I still act according to my values as a person and as a professional.
	13. I am aware of tension in my body when work is stressful.
	14. I don't have to control my negative thoughts and feelings at work to do a good job.
	15. When I'm frustrated with a patient, I am still able to provide the same quality of care as I do for a patient I like.
	16. I don't ruminate excessively about a difficult medical decision after the fact.
	17. I don't avoid calling a patient back even if I know the patient is angry or unhappy with me.
	18. I am able to continue with my daily practice as usual after an interaction with an emotionally challenging patient.

	19. I use daily routines that help me stay focused, aware, and attentive to patients' needs.
	20. I don't struggle with my emotions before, during, or after I see a difficult, hostile patient.
	Total Score

Scoring Instructions: Add your responses. The sum of your twenty responses is your total score.

Interpreting Scores: Higher scores suggest greater psychological flexibility (range: 0 to 120). Remember, your scores will change over time, and you can use real behavior change strategies to raise your score.

Primary Care Provider Stress Checklist (PCP-SC)

Name: _____   Date: _____

Below is a list of specific situations that may cause stress for people working in medical settings. Rate the extent to which each situation is stressful for you *at this moment*. Use the following scale to choose your response. For example, if you find a situation "Highly Stressful," record 5 in the "Response" column, and if it is "Not Stressful" or absent for you, record 0. To get a picture of what stresses you the most, follow the directions for scoring at the bottom of the form.

0	1	2	3	4	5	6
Not Stressful	Very Mild Stress	Mild Stress	Moderate Stress	Greater than Moderate	Highly Stressful	Extremely Stressful

INTERACTIONS WITH PATIENTS	
Response	**Stressful Situation**
	Patients who don't manage their chronic diseases. Patients who abuse or are addicted to alcohol or drugs.
	Patients who complain of chronic pain and are seeking narcotics.
	Patients who are angry and demanding.
	Patients complaining of depression, anxiety, and other common psychological problems.
	Patients who have unhealthy lifestyles (overeat, under-exercise, overwork).
	Patients who perpetrate violence or abuse on children, domestic partners, elderly relatives.
Category Total	

PRACTICE MANAGEMENT	
Response	**Stressful Situation**
	My schedule is too tight to address more than one or two problems.
	Patients wait too long because of office work-flow problems.
	Chart and other important records information is not available.
	Lack of immediate access to information about clinical guidelines.
	Not enough time to address multiple medical and mental health problems in complex patients.
	Dealing with interruptions and other annoyances during clinic/workday.
Category Total	

ADMINISTRATIVE ISSUES	
Response	**Stressful Situation**
	Unrealistic productivity standards from my employer/ practice partners.
	Billing and coding processes are hard to understand and/ or time consuming.
	Preauthorization for patient procedures and medications.
	Support-staff turnover and lack of training impact practice flow.
	Communicating with managers who seem to be more concerned with "numbers" than with quality of care.
	Work hours are too long.
	Category Total

EDUCATION/LEARNING	
Response	**Stressful Situation**
	Learning new procedures.
	Being required to make medical decisions with limited information.
	Lack of opportunity to reflect on knowledge before applying it.
	Lack of opportunity to discuss medical issues with colleagues.
	Difficulty applying new guideline information during visits with patients.
	Keeping up with new medical information.
	Category Total

RELATIONSHIPS WITH COLLEAGUES	
Response	**Stressful Situation**
	Communication difficulties with specialists.
	Strained or nonexistent communication with mental health clinicians.
	Lack of support from colleagues for work–home balance.
	Dealing with colleagues who make medical errors.
	Working with unmotivated colleagues in a team setting.
	Feeling isolated.
	Category Total
BALANCE BETWEEN WORK AND THE "REST OF LIFE"	
Response	**Stressful Situation**
	Lack of support of my medical career from friends and/or family.
	Not eating a healthy diet and exercising regularly.
	Missing family activities and occasions because of work demands.
	Difficulties taking time to see or make friends.
	Not finding time to do little things that give me pleasure.
	Continuing to think about medical issues after work hours.
	Category Total

Scoring Instructions:

1. Record the sum of your responses to each of the PCP-SC areas in the "Total" column. Then transfer these scores to the table below.

2. Divide each score in the "Total" column by the number indicated in the "Divide by" column (this number represents the maximum level of stress

for that area). For example, if you have a "Total" of 30 for "Interactions with Patients," you will get a .71 when you divide by 42.

3. To calculate the "Stress Score," multiply the score that results from dividing the "Total" score by the "Divide by" number and then multiply by 100. For example, you would multiply .71 by 100 to obtain a "Stress Score" of 71.

4. Record "Stress Scores" for each category in the "Stress Score" column. Stress scores will range from 0 to 100, with 0 suggesting no stress and 100 indicating maximum stress.

5. To calculate your total "PCP-SC Score," sum the scores in the "Total" column, divide by 222, and then multiply by 100. Like the "Stress Score" for each category, the "PCP-SC score" will be between 0 and 100, with 0 suggesting no stress and 100 indicating maximum stress.

Remember, your scores will change over time and you can use ACT strategies to address areas that contribute most to stress in your medical career at this time.

PCP-SC Source of Stress	Category Total	Divide By	Stress Score
Interactions with Patients		42	
Practice Management		36	
Administrative Issues		36	
Education/Learning		36	
Relationships with Colleagues		36	
Balance Between Work and the "Rest of Life"		36	
Total PCP-SC Score		222	

Interpreting Scores: Higher scores indicate greater stress in both individual Stress scores and the Total PCP-SC Score. Remember, you can lower your scores by applying real behavioral change strategies. See chapter 11 for specific ideas.

APPENDIX D

Real Behavior Change Interviewing—The Three-T and Workability Questions

Time	When did this start? How often does it happen? Does it happen at a particular time? What happens just before the problem? Immediately after the problem? How long does it last when it is present? Is it here all the time or is it episodic?
Trigger	What do you think is causing the problem? Is there anything that, or anyone who, seems to set it off?
Trajectory	What has this problem been like over time? Have there been times when it was less of a concern? More of a concern? Has it been getting better or worse over time? How about recently?
Workability Questions	What have you tried to cope with this problem? How have these strategies worked over time? Are you getting the kind of results you want? When you use this strategy, are you getting some accidental negative results in other areas?

Real Behavior Change Interviewing—The Love, Work, Play, and Health Questions

Love	Where do you live?
	With whom?
	How long have you been there?
	Are things okay at your home?
	Do you have loving relationships with your family or friends?
Work	Do you work? Study?
	If yes, what is your work? Study?
	Do you enjoy it?
	If no, are you looking for work?
	If no, how do you support yourself?

Play	What do you do for fun?
	For relaxation?
	For connecting with people in your neighborhood or community?
	Do you have friends? What do you do together?
Health	Do you use tobacco, alcohol, or illegal drugs?
	Do you exercise on a regular basis for your health?
	Do you eat well? Sleep well?

Six Core Processes— Psychological Flexibility

Experience the
Present Moment

Accept TEAMS
and Focus on
Action

Psychological

Flexibility

and

Vitality

Strengthen
Connection with
Values

Step Back from
TEAMS and
Unworkable Rules

Sustain
Value-Consistent
Action

Use Observer Self
to See Limiting
Self-Stories

APPENDIX G

Core Process Assessment Tool (CPAT)

Six Core Processes: Psychological Rigidity	Patient Rating Today	Six Core Processes: Psychological Flexibility
Lives in the past or future		Experiences the present moment
Disconnected from values		Strongly connected with values
Engages in impulsive, self-defeating action or inaction		Sustains value-consistent action
Stuck in limiting self-stories		Uses observer self to see limiting self-stories
Stuck in TEAMS and unworkable rules		Steps back from TEAMS and unworkable rules
Actively avoids TEAMS		Accepts TEAMS and focuses on action

How to Use the CPAT to Conceptualize and Plan Treatment:

1. Mark an "X" for each of the six core processes to indicate the patient's current position on a continuum ranging from rigid to flexible.

2. An "X" on the left-hand side indicates rigidity, while an "X" on the right indicates flexibility. If you like, you can use a rating scale ranging from 0 (most rigid) to 10 (most flexible) that will allow you to calculate a total flexibility score (ranging from 0 to 60).

3. Select one or more processes to target in a patient visit.

4. Refer to the Real Behavior Change Pocket Guide (appendix H) to choose one or more techniques for the process you plan to target.

5. You may choose a process that represents a patient's strength or weakness. In some cases, you will sense that a patient needs to gain strength in one process before working on another. For example, a patient with a history of trauma may benefit from learning more about how to experience the present moment before learning skills that help him or her sustain value-consistent action.

6. Remember that you will often help a patient in several processes, even if you target only one, because all of the processes overlap.

7. Using the CPAT on a regular basis provides you with a global impression of the patient's relative strengths and weaknesses and a sense of the patient's progress over time.

Real Behavior Change Pocket Guide

Six Core Processes: Psychological Flexibility	Technique	Demonstration Chapter
Experience the Present Moment		
	Time Line	8 (anxiety, depression)
	Three (or Five) Senses	8 (anxiety, depression)
	Balloon Breath	9 (trauma)
Strengthen Connection with Values		
	Retirement Party/ Tombstone	11 (provider wellness)
	Bull's-Eye: Value–Behavior Identification	5 (chronic disease)
	Bull's-Eye: Value–Behavior Discrepancy	5 (chronic disease)

	Bull's-Eye: Professional and Personal Values Assessment	11 (provider wellness)
Sustain Value-Consistent Action		
	You Are Not Responsible; You Are Response Able	9 (trauma)
	All Hands on Deck	7 (chronic pain)
	Bull's-Eye: Action Steps	5 (chronic disease) 6 (substance abuse) 9 (trauma)
	Burnout Prevention and Recovery Plan	11 (provider wellness)
Use Observer Self to See Limiting Self-Stories		
	What Are Your Self-Stories?	9 (trauma)
	Be a Witness	6 (substance abuse) 9 (trauma)
	Circles of Self	8 (anxiety, depression)
	Miracle Question	8 (anxiety, depression)
Step Back from TEAMS and Unworkable Rules		
	Playing with Sticky TEAMS	5 (chronic disease)
	TEAMS Sheet	7 (chronic pain)
	Velcro	11 (provider wellness)
	Clouds in the Sky	11 (provider wellness)
Accept TEAMS and Focus on Action		

	Eagle Perspective	7 (chronic pain)
	Book Chapter	5 (chronic disease)
	Rule of Mental Events	6 (substance abuse)
	Lose Control of Your Feelings, Gain Control of Your Life	6 (substance abuse)

Note: The Bull's-Eye Worksheet provides a structure for using all three of the Bull's-Eye intervention components (Value Identification, Value–Behavior Discrepancy, and Action Steps) with patients on an ongoing basis.

How to Use the Real Behavior Change Pocket Guide:

1. Print a copy of the pocket guide and keep it on a clipboard or in another place where you can find it easily at your clinic.

2. Refer to the brief descriptions of the techniques in chapter 4 as needed.

3. Study applications of the techniques in the case examples in the chapters indicated on the pocket guide.

4. Practice a technique (ideally with a colleague, a preceptor, or a friend) prior to using it.

5. When charting, indicate the process you targeted and the intervention you used.

6. With practice, you will become skillful at using a variety of techniques for each process.

Patient Education—
Bull's-Eye Worksheet

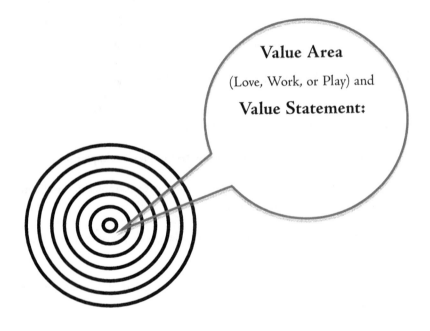

Value Area

(Love, Work, or Play) and

Value Statement:

1	2	3	4	5	6	7
Not Consistent	Slightly Consistent	Somewhat Consistent	Consistent	Remarkably Consistent	Very Consistent	Bull's-Eye!

Action Steps:

1.

2.

3.

Guide for Using the Bull's-Eye Worksheet

1. Ask the patient to choose love, work, or play as a focus for a short discussion about values. Have the patient explain what's important to him in each area of life.

2. Listen closely, reflect what you heard, then write a statement on the Bull's-Eye Worksheet using the (global, abstract) words the patient used when talking about the value.

3. Explain to the patient that the bull's-eye on the target represents hitting your value target on a daily basis (and explain that most of us fall far short of that on a day-to-day basis, but knowing what the target is helps us make choices, set goals, and implement plans).

4. Ask the patient to mark an "X" on the target (or choose a number, with 0 being most distant from values and 7 being completely consistent with values) to indicate how close to the bull's-eye value statement her behavior has come over the past two weeks.

5. Ask the patient to plan one or more specific behavior experiments for the next two weeks that the patient believes will make his behavior more value consistent (closer to the bull's-eye target).

6. If time allows, rate the patient's current functioning level in one or more core areas on the CPAT (appendix G). This will provide a baseline against which you can judge the impact of the Bull's-Eye Worksheet.

7. If time allows, choose a core process area and a corresponding technique from the Real Behavior Change Pocket Guide (appendix H) to use in the visit.

8. At follow-up, ask the patient to re-rate value consistency (see step 4, above) and then to identify barriers to engaging in behaviors planned in the prior visit. Often, identifying barriers will point to the core process the patient needs to address in that visit to develop greater flexibility.

Provider Tool—Retirement Party Worksheet

Instructions: For each of the following four life areas, describe your core values. For example, if you were at your own retirement party, what would you like to hear other people say about what you stood for, the mark you left generally, what your behavior over the years demonstrated about your personal beliefs?

Studying or Practicing Medicine (for example, your efforts to learn or practice):

Professional Relationships:

Teaching Medicine (for example, your efforts to prepare others for medical careers):

Balancing Professional and Private Lives:

Provider Tool—Bull's-Eye Professional and Personal Values Assessment

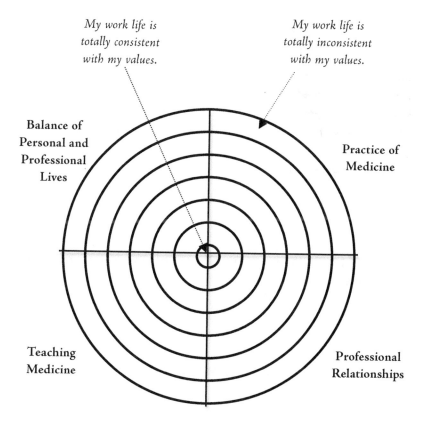

My work life is totally consistent with my values.

My work life is totally inconsistent with my values.

Balance of Personal and Professional Lives

Practice of Medicine

Teaching Medicine

Professional Relationships

Instructions: Place an "X" or draw a star in each of the four quadrants to represent the degree to which you have been living according to your values in each area during the past month.

APPENDIX L

Burnout Prevention and Recovery Plan

To help reduce your risk of burnout, describe specific behaviors you intend to use, when you will use them, and how often for each of the following four skill areas. Try to respond to at least two areas initially and add more plans later. The more specific your plan, the more likely you are to follow it!

Practice of Acceptance:

Practice of Mindfulness (for example, present-moment awareness, contacting observer self):

Practice of Contact with Personal Values:

Practice of Value-Consistent Daily Action:

References

Beardsley, R. S., Gardocki, G. J., Larson, D. B., & Hidalgo, J. (1988). Prescribing of psychotropic medication by primary care physicians and psychiatrists. *Archives of General Psychiatry, 45*(12), 1117–1119.

Beck, J. S. (1995). *Cognitive therapy: Basics and beyond.* New York: The Guilford Press.

Blackledge, J. T. (2003). An introduction to relational frame theory: Basics and applications. *The Behavior Analyst Today, 3*(4), 421–433.

Bond, F. W., Hayes, S. C., Baer, R. A., Carpenter, K. M., Orcutt, H. K., Waltz, T., et al. (2010). *Preliminary psychometric properties of the Acceptance and Action Questionnaire II: A revised measure of psychological flexibility and acceptance.*

Branstetter-Rost, A., Cushing, C., & Douleh, T. (2009). Personal values and pain tolerance: Does a values intervention add to acceptance? *Journal of Pain, 10*(8), 887–892.

Bureau of Justice Statistics (2007). *Criminal victimization in the United States, 2007: Statistical tables.* Washington, DC: United States Government Printing Office. http://bjs.ojp.usdoj.gov/index.cfm?ty=pbse&sid=58.

Center, C., Davis, M., Detre, T., Ford, D. E., Hansbrough, W., Hendin, H., et al. (2003). Confronting depression and suicide in physicians: A consensus statement. *Journal of the American Medical Association, 289*(23), 3161–3166.

Ciarrochi, J., Forgas, J. P., & Mayer, J. D. (eds.) (2006). *Emotional intelligence in everyday life: A scientific inquiry* (2nd ed.). New York: Psychology Press.

Ciarrochi, J., & Mayer, J. D. (eds.) (2007). *Applying emotional intelligence: A practitioner's guide* (1st ed.). New York: Psychology Press.

Conway, T., Hu, T. C., Warshaw, C., Kim, P., & Bullon, A. (1995). Violence victims' perception of functioning and well-being: A survey from an urban public hospital walk-in clinic. *Journal of the National Medical Association, 87*(6), 407–413.

Dahl, J., Wilson, K. G., & Nilsson, A. (2004). Acceptance and commitment therapy and the treatment of persons at risk for long-term disability resulting from stress and pain symptoms: A preliminary randomized trial. *Behavior Therapy, 35*(4), 785–801.

Deckard, G., Meterko, M., & Field, D. (1994). Physician burnout: An examination of personal, professional, and organizational relationships. *Medical Care, 32*(7), 745–754.

Desai, R. A., Harpaz-Rotem, I., Najavits, L. M., & Rosenheck, R. A. (2008). Impact of the seeking safety program on clinical outcomes among homeless female veterans with psychiatric disorders. *Psychiatric Services, 59*(9), 1–25.

de Shazer, S. (1988). *Clues: Investigating solutions in brief therapy.* New York: W. W. Norton & Company.

Dick, B. D., & Rashiq, S. (2007). Disruption of attention and working memory traces in individuals with chronic pain. *Anesthesia and Analgesia, 104*(5), 1223–1229.

Dunbar-Jacob, J., & Mortimer-Stephens, M. K. (2001). Treatment adherence in chronic disease. *Journal of Clinical Epidemiology, 54*(Suppl. 1), S57–S60.

Dyrbye, L. N., Thomas, M. R., Huntington, J. L., Lawson, K. L., Novotny P. J., Sloan, J. A., et al. (2006). Personal life events and medical student burnout: A multicenter study. *Academic Medicine, 81*(4), 374–384.

D'Zurilla, T. J., & Nezu, A. M. (1999). *Problem-solving therapy: A social competence approach to clinical intervention* (2nd ed.). New York: Springer Publishing Company.

Ellis, A. (2001). *Overcoming destructive beliefs, feelings, and behaviors: New directions for rational emotive behavior therapy.* Amherst, NY: Prometheus Books.

European General Practice Research Network Burnout Study Group (2008). Burnout in European family doctors: The EGPRN study. *Family Practice, 25*(4), 245–265.

Fahrenkopf, A. M., Sectish, T. C., Barger, L. K., Sharek, P. J., Lewin, D., Chiang, V. W., et al. (2008). Rates of medication errors among depressed and burnt out residents: Prospective cohort study. *British Medical Journal, 336*(7642), 488–491.

Forman, E. M., Herbert, J. D., Moitra, E., Yeomans, P. D., & Geller, P. A. (2007). A randomized controlled effectiveness trial of acceptance and commitment therapy and cognitive therapy for anxiety and depression. *Behavior Modification, 31*(6), 772–799.

Forsyth, J. P., & Eifert, G. H. (2007). *The mindfulness and acceptance workbook for anxiety: A guide to breaking free from anxiety, phobias & worry using acceptance and commitment therapy.* Oakland, CA: New Harbinger Publications.

Gifford, E. V., Kohlenberg, B. S., Hayes, S. C., Antonuccio, D. O., Piasecki, M. M., Rasmussen-Hall, M. L., & Palm, K. M. (2004). Acceptance-based treatment for smoking cessation. *Behavior Therapy, 35*(4), 689–705.

Gregg, J. A., Callaghan, G. M., & Hayes, S. C. (2007). *The diabetes lifestyle book: Facing your fears and making changes for a long and healthy life.* Oakland, CA: New Harbinger Publications.

Gregg, J. A., Callaghan, G. M., Hayes, S. C., & Glenn-Lawson, J. L. (2007). Improving diabetes self-management through acceptance, mindfulness, and values: A randomized controlled trial. *Journal of Consulting and Clinical Psychology, 75*(2), 336–343.

Grossman, P., Niemann, L., Schmidt, S., & Walach, H. (2004). Mindfulness-based stress reduction and health benefits: A meta-analysis. *Journal of Psychosomatic Research, 57*(1), 35–43.

Hayes, S. C., Barnes-Holmes, D., & Roche, B. (eds.) (2001). *Relational frame theory: A post-Skinnerian account of human language and cognition.* New York: Kluwer Academic/Plenum Publishers.

Hayes, S. C., Bissett, R., Roget, N., Padilla, M., Kohlenberg, B. S., Fisher, G., et al. (2004). The impact of acceptance and commitment training and multicultural training on the stigmatizing attitudes and professional burnout of substance abuse counselors. *Behavior Therapy, 35*(4), 821–835.

Hayes, S. C., Luoma, J. B., Bond, F. W., Masuda, A., & Lillis, J. (2006). Acceptance and commitment therapy: Model, processes, and outcomes. *Behaviour Research and Therapy, 44*(1), 1–25.

Hayes, S. C., Strosahl, K. D., & Wilson, K. G. (1999). *Acceptance and commitment therapy: An experiential approach to behavior change.* New York: The Guilford Press.

Hayes, S. C., Strosahl, K., Wilson, K. G., Bissett, R. T., Pistorello, J., Toarmino, D., et al. (2004). Measuring experiential avoidance: A preliminary test of a working model. *Psychological Record, 54*(4), 553–578.

Hayes, S. C., Wilson, K. G., Gifford, E. V., Follette, V. M., & Strosahl, K. (1996). Emotional avoidance and behavioral disorders: A functional dimensional approach to diagnosis and treatment. *Journal of Consulting and Clinical Psychology, 64*(6), 1152–1168.

Hayes, S. C., Wilson, K. G., Gifford, E. V., Bissett, R., Piasecki, M., Batten, S. V., et al. (2004). A preliminary trial of twelve-step facilitation and acceptance and commitment therapy with polysubstance-abusing methadone-maintained opiate addicts. *Behavior Therapy, 35*, 667–688.

Katon, W., Robinson, P., von Korff, M., Lin, E., Bush, T., Ludman, E., et al. (1996). A multifaceted intervention to improve treatment of depression in primary care. *Archives of General Psychiatry, 53*(10), 924–932.

Katon, W. J., Roy-Byrne, P., Russo, J., & Cowley, D. (2002). Cost effectiveness and cost offset of a collaborative care intervention for primary care patients with panic disorder. *Archives of General Psychiatry, 59*(12), 1098–1104.

Kessler, R. C., Berglund, P., Demler, O., Jin, R., Merikangas, K. R., & Walters, E. E. (2005). Lifetime prevalence and age-of-onset distributions of DSM-IV disorders in the National Comorbidity Survey Replication. *Archives of General Psychiatry, 62*(6), 593–602.

Koss, M. P., Koss, P. G., & Woodruff, W. J. (1991). Deleterious effects of criminal victimization on women's health and medical utilization. *Archives of Internal Medicine, 151*(2), 342–349.

Landon, B. E., Reschovsky, J. D., Pham, H. H., & Blumenthal, D. (2006). Leaving medicine: The consequences of physician dissatisfaction. *Medical Care, 44*(3), 234–242.

Last, J. M. (1988). *A dictionary of epidemiology.* New York: Oxford University Press.

Lee, F. J., Brown, J. B., & Stewart, M. (2009). Exploring family physician stress: Helpful strategies. *Canadian Family Physician, 55*(3), 288–289.

Lee, F. J., Stewart, M., & Brown, J. B. (2008). Stress, burnout, and strategies for reducing them: What's the situation among Canadian family physicians? *Canadian Family Physician, 54*(2), 234–235.

Leiter, M. & Maslach, C. (2009). Nurse turnover: The mediating role of burnout. *Journal of Nursing Management, 17,* 331–339.

Linzer, M., Baier Manwell, L., Williams, E. S., Bobula, J. A., Brown, R. L., Varkey, A. B., et al. (2009). Working conditions in primary care: Physician reactions and care quality. *Annals of Internal Medicine, 151*(1), 28–36.

Linzer, M., Gerrity, M., Douglas, J. A., McMurray, J. E., Williams, E. S., & Konrad, T. R. (2002). Physician stress: Results from the physician worklife study. *Stress and Health, 18*(1), 37–42.

Losa Iglesias, M. E., Becerro de Bengoa Vallejo, R., & Salvadores Fuentes, P. (2010). The relationship between experiential avoidance and burnout syndrome in critical care nurses: A cross-sectional questionnaire survey. *International Journal of Nursing Studies, 47*(1):30–37.

Lundgren, T., Dahl, J., Yardi, N., & Melin, L. (2008). Acceptance and commitment therapy and yoga for drug-refractory epilepsy: A randomized controlled trial. *Epilepsy and Behavior, 13*(1), 102–108.

Martini, S., Arfken, C. L., & Balon, R. (2006). Comparison of burnout among medical residents before and after the implementation of work hours limits. *Academic Psychiatry, 30*(4), 352–355.

Maslach, C., Jackson, S., & Leiter, M. P. (1996). *The Maslach Burnout Inventory* (3rd ed.) Palo Alto: Consulting Psychologists Press.

Maslach, C., Schaufeli, W. B., & Leiter, M. P. (2001). Job burnout. *Annual Review of Psychology, 52*, 397–422. doi:10.1146/annurev.psych.52.1.397

McCaig, L. F., & Burt, C. W. (2004). National Hospital Ambulatory Medical Care Survey: 2002 Emergency department summary. *Advance data from vital and health statistics, 340*. Hyattsville, MD: National Center for Health Statistics.

McCracken, L. M., & Eccleston, C. (2003). Coping or acceptance: What to do about chronic pain? *Pain, 105*(1–2), 197–204.

Meresman, J. F., Hunkeler, E. M., Hargreaves, W. A., Kirsch, A. J., Robinson, P., Green, A., et al. (2003). A case report: Implementing a nurse tele-care program for treating depression in primary care. *Psychiatric Quarterly, 74*(1), 61–73.

Miller, W. R., & Rollnick, S. (2002). *Motivational interviewing: Preparing people for change* (2nd ed.). New York: The Guilford Press.

Nampiaparampil, D. E. (2008). Prevalence of chronic pain after traumatic brain injury: A systematic review. *Journal of the American Medical Association, 300*(6), 711–719.

Patterson, J. E., Peek, C. J., Heinrich, R. L., Bischoff, R. J., & Scherger, J. (2002). *Mental health professionals in medical settings: A primer.* New York: W. W. Norton and Company.

Platt, F. W., & Gordon, G. H. (1999). *Field guide to the difficult patient interview.* Philadelphia: Lippincott Williams & Wilkins.

Powers, M. B., Zum Vörde Sive Vörding, M. B., & Emmelkamp, P. M. (2009). Acceptance and commitment therapy: A meta-analytic review. *Psychotherapy and Psychosomatics, 78*(2), 73–80.

Rafferty, J. P., Lemkau, J. P., Purdy, R. R., & Rudisill, J. R. (1986). Validity of the Maslach Burnout Inventory for family practice physicians. *Journal of Clinical Psychology, 42*(3), 488–493.

Ratanawongsa, N., Roter, D., Beach, M. C., Laird, S. L., Larson, S. M., Carson, K. A., et al. (2008). Physician burnout and patient-physician communication during primary care encounters. *Journal of General Internal Medicine, 23*(10), 1581–1588.

Ratanawongsa, N., Wright, S. M., & Carrese, J. A. (2007). Well-being in residency: A time for temporary imbalance? *Medical Education, 41*(3), 273–280.

Robinson, P. (1996). *Living life well: New strategies for hard times.* Reno, NV: Context Press.

Robinson, P., Wischman, C., & del Vento, A. (1996). *Treating depression in primary care: A manual for primary care and mental health providers.* Reno, NV: Context Press.

Robinson, P. J., & Reiter, J. T. (2007). *Behavioral consultation and primary care: A guide to integrating services.* New York: Springer Science+Business Media.

Sartorius, N., Ustün, T. B., Lecrubier, Y., & Wittchen, H. U. (1996). Depression cormorbid with anxiety: Results from the WHO study on psychological disorders in primary health care. *British Journal of Psychiatry Supplement, 30,* 38–43.

Schernhammer, E. S., & Colditz, G. A. (2004). Suicide rates among physicians: A quantitative and gender assessment (meta-analysis). *American Journal of Psychiatry, 161*(12), 2295–2302.

Schneider Institutes for Health Policy (2001). *Substance abuse: The nation's number one health problem—Key indicators for policy update.* Prepared for the Robert Wood Johnson Foundation, Princeton, NJ. Waltham, MA: Schneider Institutes for Health Policy, Brandeis University.

Skinner, B. F. (1950). Are theories of learning necessary? *Psychological Review, 57*(4), 193–216.

Skinner, B. F. (1989). The origins of cognitive thought. *American Psychologist, 44*(1), 13–18.

Stein, M. B., McQuaid, J. R., Pedrelli, P., Lenox, R., & McCahill, M. E. (2000). Posttraumatic stress disorder in the primary care medical setting. *General Hospital Psychiatry, 22*(4), 261–265.

Strosahl, K. D., & Robinson, P. J. (2008). *The acceptance and mindfulness workbook for depression: Using acceptance and commitment therapy to move through depression and create a life worth living.* Oakland, CA: New Harbinger Publications.

Stuart, M. R., & Lieberman, J. A. (2002). *The fifteen-minute hour: Practical therapeutic interventions in primary care* (3rd ed.). New York: Elsevier Press.

Törneke, N., & Luoma, J. B. (2009, July). *Relational frame theory: Basic concepts and clinical applications.* Workshop at the Association for Contextual Behavioval Science World Conference III, Enschede, Netherlands.

Törneke, N. (2010). *Learning RFT.* Oakland, CA: New Harbinger Publications.

Tunks, E. R., Crook, J., & Weir, R. (2008). Epidemiology of chronic pain with psychological cormorbidity: Prevalence, risk, course, and prognosis. *Canadian Journal of Psychiatry, 53*(4), 224–234.

Turner, E. H., Matthews, A. M., Linardatos, E., Tell, R. A., & Rosenthal, R. (2008). Selective publication of antidepressant trials and its influence on apparent efficacy. *New England Journal of Medicine, 358*(3), 252–260.

United States Preventive Services Task Force (2009). Screening for depression in adults. Retrieved September 14, 2010, from http://www.uspreventiveservicestaskforce.org/uspstf/uspsabrecs.htm.

Unützer, J. (2007). Clinical practice: Late-life depression. *New England Journal of Medicine, 357*(22), 2269–2276.

Vieweg, W. V., Julius, D. A., Fernandez, A., Beatty-Brooks, M., Hettema, J. M., & Pandurangi, A. K. (2006). Posttraumatic stress disorder: Clinical features, pathophysiology, and treatment. *American Journal of Medicine, 119*(5), 383–388.

Vowles, K. E., McNeil, D. W., Gross, R. T., McDaniel, M. L., Mouse, A., Bates, M., et al. (2007). Effects of pain acceptance and pain control strategies on physical impairment in individuals with chronic low back pain. *Behavior Therapy, 38*(4), 412–425.

Walker, E. A., Katon, W., Russo, J., Ciechanowski, P., Newman, E., & Wagner, A. W. (2003). Health care costs associated with posttraumatic stress disorder symptoms in women. *Archives of General Psychiatry, 60*(4), 369–374.

Wang, P. S., Lane, M., Olfson, M., Pincus, H. A., Wells, K. B., & Kessler, R. C. (2005). Twelve-month use of mental health services in the United States: Results from the National Comorbidity Survey Replication. *Archives of General Psychiatry, 62*(6), 590–592.

Watson, J. B. (1913). Psychology as the behaviorist views it. *Psychological Review, 20,* 158–177.

Wells, K. B., Steward, A., Hays, R. D., Burnam, M. A., Rogers, W., Daniels, M., et al. (1989). The functioning and well-being of depressed patients: Results from the Medical Outcomes Study. *Journal of the American Medical Association, 262*(7), 914–919.

Wegner, D. M., Schneider, D. J., Carter III, S. R., & White, T. L. (1987). Paradoxical effects of thought suppression. *Journal of Personality and Social Psychology, 53*(1), 5–13.

West, C. P., Tan, A. D., Habermann, T. M., Sloan, J. A., & Shanafelt, T. D. (2009). Association of resident fatigue and distress with perceived medical errors. *Journal of the American Medical Association, 302*(12), 1294–1299.

Wolpe, J. (1958). *Psychotherapy by reciprocal inhibition.* Stanford, CA: Stanford University Press.

Zettle, R. D., & Rains, J. C. (1989). Group cognitive and contextual therapies in treatment of depression. *Journal of Clinical Psychology, 45*(3), 436–445.

Patricia J. Robinson, PhD, is director of training for Mountainview Consulting Group and recipient of the American Psychological Association's 2009 Innovative Practice Award. She has worked as a health care provider and researcher for more than thirty years. Currently, she consults with and provides training for health care systems all over the world. She is coauthor of *Behavioral Consultation and Primary Care*.

Debra A. Gould, MD, MPH, is associate clinical professor in the department of family medicine at the University of Washington School of Medicine, and has taught medical students and family medicine residents for more than twenty years. She practices at Central Washington Family Medicine Residency Program in Yakima, WA. Her interests include evidence-based practice, mental health issues in primary care, community medicine, practice-based research, and physician wellness.

Kirk D. Strosahl, PhD, is clinical assistant professor in the department of family medicine at the University of Washington School of Medicine. He practices at Central Washington Family Medicine Residency Program in Yakima, WA, and is cofounder of acceptance and commitment therapy. He has worked for over two decades in primary care medical settings, collaborating with health care providers of all disciplines and training family medicine residents.

Index

A

abuse: victims of, 155-156. *See also* trauma interventions

acceptance: chronic disease patients and, 97; chronic pain patients and, 121-122; explanation of, 56; provider wellness and, 202-203; techniques for enhancing, 57-58, 79; willingness and, 56-57

Acceptance and Action Questionnaire II (AAQ-II), 7, 182, 205-206

ACT (acceptance and commitment therapy), 3; burnout prevention and, 181; diabetes patients and, 87-88; listening based on, 63-64; occupational stress and, 5-6; research on primary care and, 3-5

action: focusing on, 56-58, 79; impulsive or self-defeating, 32-33; value- consistent, 50-52, 78-79

action steps, 51-52; alcohol/drug abuse interventions and, 116, 117; chronic disease patients and, 98-100; chronic pain patients and, 129, 134; provider wellness interventions and, 201-203; trauma interventions and, 171-172

activities of daily living (ADLs), 90

addiction, substance abuse, 104

alcohol/drug abuse interventions, 103-118; ACT perspective on, 104; action steps, 116, 117; Be a Witness exercise, 114-115; behavior-change interview, 106-112; Bull's-Eye Worksheet, 115-116; case example of, 105-117; follow-up care for, 117; Lose Control of Your Feelings, Gain Control of Your Life technique, 112-113;

observer self and, 114-115; overview of, 103-105; planning and providing treatment, 112-116; Rule of Mental Events technique, 114; summary of, 117-118; values connection, 115-116

All Hands on Deck game, 51, 132-133

antidepressants: chronic pain treatment using, 120; controlling mood states with, 137-138

anxiety: characteristics of, 140; medications for, 137-138; prevalence of, 138

anxiety and depression interventions, 137-154; behavior-change interview, 143-145; case example of, 142-153; Circles of Self exercise, 149-152; CPAT used in, 145-146; financial impact of, 138-139; follow-up care for, 149-152; Living Life Well class, 152-153; medications and, 137-138; Miracle Question technique, 148-149; mood continuum and, 139-140; observer self and, 149-152; overview of, 137-141; planning and providing treatment, 145-149; present-moment experience in, 146-149; summary of, 153-154; Three (or Five) Senses exercise, 147-148; Time Line technique, 148. *See also* anxiety; depression

appetitive control, 30

approach-oriented strategies, 42, 43

assessment: burnout risk, 182-184; professional and personal values, 197-199; tools used for, 7, 74-76, 182; workability, 42-44

associations, 23-24

aversive control, 30

avoidance: behavioral, 32-33; experiential, 35

avoidance-based strategies, 42, 43

B

Balloon Breath exercise, 47-48, 165-166

Be a Witness technique, 53; alcohol/drug abuse interventions and, 114-115; trauma interventions and, 166-168

behavior analysis, 13

behavior change: ACT approach to, 26; creating a context for, 39-59; interviewing for, 62-74; problem of, 2-3; reason giving and, 41; tools for creating, 7, 62, 64-74; unworkable agenda of, 41-42; workability and, 42-44

behavioral approaches, 11-14

behavioral avoidance, 32-33

behavioral health (BH) providers, 122

behavioral health consultant (BHC), 5, 123

behavior-change interviews: alcohol/drug abuse interventions and, 106-112; anxiety and depression interventions and, 143-145; chronic disease interventions and, 90-94; Love, Work, Play, and Health questions for, 71-74, 216-217; overview of tools for, 62, 64-74; Three-T and Workability Questions for, 65-71, 215; trauma interventions and, 159-164
behavior–value discrepancy, 49-50, 97
biomedical approach, 15-16
blame and fault, 50-51, 169-170
Book Chapter technique, 57, 97
Breath, Balloon, 47-48, 165-166
Buddha, 119
Bull's-Eye Professional and Personal Values Assessment: copy of form, 227; provider wellness and, 197-199
Bull's-Eye Worksheet, 7, 80-82; acceptance of TEAMS and, 58; action steps indicated on, 51-52; alcohol/drug abuse interventions and, 115-116; chronic disease interventions and, 95-97, 98-100; chronic pain interventions and, 129, 133-134; copy of form, 81, 224-225; guidelines for using, 82, 225; identifying values using, 48, 49, 95-96; illustrated example of, 81; printing and laminating, 80, 83; Professional

and Personal Values Assessment, 197-199, 227; provider wellness interventions and, 197-199; trauma interventions and, 170-171; value–behavior discrepancy and, 49-50, 97
burnout, 177-191; assessing risk of, 182-184; case example of, 184-189; components of, 178-179; consequences of, 180; definition of, 178; Love, Work, Play, and Health Questions, 186-187; PCP-AAQ survey tool, 182, 183, 185; PCP-SC survey tool, 182, 183-184, 186; prevalence of, 177-178; prevention of, 52, 181, 202-203; risk factors for, 5-6, 179-180; summary of, 189-190; Three-T and Workability Questions, 187-189. *See also* provider wellness interventions
Burnout Prevention and Recovery Plan, 52; copy of form, 228; provider wellness and, 202-203
buying thoughts, 55

C

case conceptualization, 7
case examples: of alcohol/drug abuse interventions, 105-117; of anxiety and depression interventions, 142-153; of burnout in primary care providers, 184-189; of chronic disease interventions, 89-101; of chronic pain interventions,

123-124; of provider wellness interventions, 195-203; of trauma interventions, 158-172

change. *See* behavior change

chronic disease interventions, 87-101; accepting difficult TEAMS, 97; ACT diabetes workshop, 87-88; action steps, 98-100; behavior-change interview, 90-94; Book Chapter technique, 97; Bull's-Eye Worksheet, 95-97, 98-100; case example of, 89-101; follow-up care for, 100-101; overview of, 87-89; planning and providing treatment, 94-100; Playing with Sticky TEAMS, 94-95; summary of, 101; values connection, 95-97

chronic pain interventions, 119-135; accepting painful TEAMS, 126; action steps, 129, 134; All Hands on Deck game, 132-133; Bull's-Eye Worksheet, 129, 133-134; case example of, 123-124; Eagle Perspective technique, 126; modeling willingness in, 121; overview of, 119-122; Pain and Quality of Life Pathway program, 122, 123, 124-125, 130-134; planning and providing treatment, 124-134; power of acceptance in, 121-122; psychological factors in, 119, 120-121; sample P&QOL class agenda, 130-131; summary

of, 134-135; TEAMS Sheet technique, 127-129

Circles of Self exercise, 54, 149-152

Clouds in the Sky exercise, 56, 201

cognitive behavioral therapy (CBT), 12-13

committed action, 56

compassion fatigue, 35

connection with values, 48-50, 78; alcohol/drug abuse interventions and, 115-116; chronic disease interventions and, 95-97; provider wellness interventions and, 195-199, 203; trauma interventions and, 170-171

contextual approach, 16-17; ACT applied as, 26; TEAMS acronym and, 20-25

control: appetitive vs. aversive, 30; weakening sense of, 179

Core Process Assessment Tool (CPAT), 7, 74-76; anxiety and depression interventions and, 145-146; copy of form, 219; guidelines for using, 220; provider wellness interventions and, 195; trauma interventions and, 164

cultural instruction, 41-42

D

defusion, 54-56, 199, 202

depersonalization, 178-179

depression: burnout and, 180; characteristics of, 139-140; chronic pain and, 119; medications for, 137-138; prevalence of, 138. *See also* anxiety and depression interventions

Desai, Rani, 157

destructive normality, principle of, 19

diabetes: ACT workshop for patients with, 87-88; case example of patient with, 89-101. *See also* chronic disease interventions

Diabetes Lifestyle Book, The (Gregg, Callaghan, and Hayes), 88, 101

directive communications, 64

disconnection from values, 32

disease, chronic. *See* chronic disease interventions

domestic violence, 103

drug use. *See* alcohol/drug abuse interventions; medications

E

Eagle Perspective technique, 57, 126

Einstein, Albert, 193

emotional exhaustion, 178

emotional intelligence (EI), 23

emotions: contextual approach to, 22-23. *See also* mood-related problems

experience: framing of, 23-24; present-moment, 46-48, 78

experiential avoidance, 35

F

fault and blame, 50-51, 169-170

Field Guide to the Difficult Patient Interview (Platt and Gordon), 2

Fifteen-Minute Hour, The (Stuart and Lieberman), 2

flexibility. *See* psychological flexibility

follow-up care: for alcohol/drug abuse patients, 117; for anxiety and depression interventions, 149-152; for chronic disease patients, 100-101; for trauma patients, 165-172

framing of experience, 23-24

functional contextualism, 16

fusion, 34

future, living in, 31, 139

H

health questions, 71, 72

health service providers. *See* primary care providers

high perspective taking, 33

holding thoughts, 55

human suffering. *See* suffering

I

imbalanced life, 180

impulsive actions, 32-33

inaction, 32-33

interventions: for alcohol/drug abuse, 103-118; for anxiety and depression, 137-154; for chronic disease, 87-101; for chronic pain, 119-135; for provider wellness, 193-204; for trauma victims, 155-173

interviewing, 62-74; basic guidelines for, 62-64; behavior-change tool kit for, 64-74; motivational, 3. *See also* behavior-change interviews

L

lack of personal accomplishment, 178, 179

language: problem solving rules and, 35; RFT model of, 13-14

Last, John, 44

Learning RFT (Törneke), 14

listening with ACT ears, 63-64

Living Life Well class, 152-153

Living Life Well: New Strategies for Hard Times (Robinson), 152

long-term action steps, 100

Lose Control of Your Feelings, Gain Control of Your Life technique, 58, 112-113

Love, Work, Play, and Health questions, 71-74; alcohol/drug abuse interventions and, 107-108; burnout risk assessment and, 186-187; chronic disease interventions and, 90-91; copy of form with, 216-217; example of using, 72-74; trauma interventions and, 160-161

love questions, 71, 72

low perspective taking, 33

lumpy TEAMS, 165

Lynch, Peter, 61

M

Maslach, Christina, 178-179

Maslach Burnout Inventory (MBI), 179

mechanism, 15-16

medical home model, 4

medical service providers. *See* primary care providers

medications: controlling mood states with, 137-138; treating chronic pain with, 120

memories, 24-25

mental fusion, 34

Milne, A. A., 137

mind-as-context model, 20-21

mind-as-machine model, 20

mindfulness practice, 203

mindfulness-based stress reduction, 3

Miracle Question technique, 54, 148-149

modeling skills, 64, 121

mood-related problems: continuum of, 139-140; financial impact of, 138-139; prevalence of, 138, 139. *See also* anxiety and depression interventions

Mother Teresa of Calcutta, 177

motivational interviewing, 3

O

observer self, 52-54, 79; alcohol/drug abuse interventions and, 114-115; anxiety and depression

interventions and, 149-152;
provider wellness interventions
and, 203; trauma interventions
and, 166-169
occupational stress, 5-6
online resources, 7, 40, 62
opioids, 120

P

pain: psychological factors related
to, 120; suffering differentiated
from, 17-18. *See also* chronic
pain interventions
Pain and Quality of Life
(P&QOL) Pathway program,
122, 123, 124-125, 130-134;
Bull's-Eye Worksheet example,
133-134; sample class agenda,
130-131
pain gate, 120
past, living in, 31, 139
pharmaceutical approach, 137-138.
See also medications
planning and providing
treatments: for alcohol/drug
abuse, 112-116; for anxiety and
depression, 145-149; for chronic
disease patients, 94-100; for
chronic pain patients, 124-134;
tools used for, 7, 62, 74-82, 83;
for trauma patients, 164
play questions, 71, 72
Playing with Sticky TEAMS
technique, 55, 94-95
plys and pliance, 32
post-traumatic stress disorder
(PTSD), 119, 156

present-moment experience,
46; anxiety and depression
interventions and, 146-149;
provider wellness interventions
and, 203; techniques to
enhance, 47-48, 78; trauma
interventions and, 165-166
primary care: alcohol/drug
abuse interventions and, 103-
118; anxiety and depression
interventions and, 137-154;
chronic disease interventions
and, 87-101; chronic pain
interventions and, 119-135;
research on ACT and, 3-5;
trauma interventions and,
155-173
primary care behavioral health
(PCBH) model, 4, 122
Primary Care Provider Acceptance
and Action Questionnaire
(PCP-AAQ), 7; burnout risk
assessment, 182, 183, 185; copy
of form, 207-209
Primary Care Provider Stress
Checklist (PCP-SC), 7; burnout
risk assessment, 182, 183-184,
186; copy of form, 210-214;
guideline for using, 7-8
primary care providers (PCPs):
ACT-based methods and, 6;
occupational stress factors for,
5-6; risk of burnout for, 177-
191; use of term, 5; wellness
interventions for, 193-204
principle of destructive normality,
19
problem solving, rules of, 35

Professional and Personal Values Assessment, 197-199
provider wellness interventions, 193-204; action steps, 201-203; Bull's-Eye Worksheet, 197-199; Burnout Prevention and Recovery Plan, 202-203; case example of, 195-203; Clouds in the Sky exercise, 201; CPAT used in, 195; overview of, 193-194; Professional and Personal Values Assessment, 197-199; Retirement Party Worksheet, 49, 195-196; summary of, 204; values connection, 195-199, 203; Velcro exercise, 56, 199-200
psychoanalysis, 11
psychological flexibility, 18, 45-58; core processes supporting, 45-58, 218; CPAT tool for assessing, 74-76; diagram of six core processes, 46, 218; pocket guide for behavior change and, 76-80; techniques for enhancing, 47-58, 76-80; vitality and, 45-46
psychological problems: alcohol/drug abuse and, 104; behavioral approaches to, 11-14; chronic pain and, 119, 120-121
psychological rigidity, 18; core processes contributing to, 30-35; CPAT tool for assessing, 74-76; TEAMS content and, 29

Q

questions: asking in interviews, 64, 65-74; Love, Work, Play, and Health, 71-74; Miracle Question technique, 54, 148-149; Three-T and Workability, 65-71

R

radical behaviorists, 13
reactive mind, 52
Real Behavior Change Pocket Guide, 7, 76-80; burnout prevention/recovery and, 202; copy of form, 78-79, 221-223; instructions on using, 80, 223
reason giving, 41
rebound effect, 19, 35
reductionism, 15
relational frame theory (RFT), 13-14
Response Able exercise, 50-51, 170
responsibility, 50-51, 170
Retirement Party Worksheet, 49; copy of form, 226; provider wellness and, 195-196
rigidity. *See* psychological rigidity
risk factors for burnout, 5-6, 179-180
role-modeling skills, 64
rule of mental events, 35, 58
Rule of Mental Events technique, 58, 114
rules: problem solving, 35; stepping back from, 54-56; stuckness in unworkable, 34;

values vs. following of, 32. *See also* unworkable rules

S

self: circles of, 54; observer, 52-54, 79
self-defeating actions, 32-33
self-fulfilling prophecy, 33
self-stories: alcohol/drug abuse interventions and, 114-115; anxiety and depression interventions and, 149-152; chronic disease interventions, 97; exercise for discussing, 53; observer self and, 52-54, 79; stuckness in, 33-34; trauma interventions and, 168-169
sensations, 25
sexual abuse: victims of, 156, 157. *See also* trauma interventions
short-term action steps: chronic disease interventions and, 99-100; trauma interventions and, 171
signaling systems, 23
Skinner, B. F., 13
slowing down, 63
social support, 179
Souza, Alfred D., 29
sticky TEAMS, 55, 94-95, 199-200
stress: ACT and occupational, 5-6; burnout risk and, 182, 183-184, 186; factors contributing to, 5-6

stuckness: core processes related to, 29-37. *See also* psychological rigidity
substance abuse interventions. *See* alcohol/drug abuse interventions
suffering: behavioral approaches to, 11-14; biomedical approach to, 15-16; contextual approach to, 16-17, 20-25; pain differentiated from, 17-18; pharmaceutical approach to, 137-138

T

TEAMS, 20-25; acceptance of, 56-58, 79; active avoidance of, 35; alcohol/drug abuse and, 112-114; chronic disease patients and, 94-95, 97, 112-114; chronic pain patients and, 126-129; playing with sticky, 55, 94-95; presentation of lumpy, 165; provider wellness and, 199-201; psychological rigidity and, 29; stepping back from, 54-56, 79, 94-95, 127-129, 199-201; stuckness in, 34
TEAMS sheet, 55, 127-129
thoughts: contextual approach to, 21-22; holding vs. buying, 55; RFT model of, 13-14
Three (or Five) Senses technique, 47, 147-148
Three-T and Workability Questions, 65-71; alcohol/drug abuse interventions and, 109-

111; anxiety and depression interventions and, 143-145; burnout risk assessment and, 187-189; chronic disease interventions and, 92-93; copy of form with, 215; example of using, 67-70; trauma interventions and, 161-164
Time Line technique, 47, 148
time questions, 66, 67
Tombstone exercise, 49, 195
toxic work culture, 179
trajectory questions, 67, 68
trauma interventions, 155-173; action steps, 171-172; Balloon Breath exercise, 165-166; Be a Witness technique, 166-168; behavior change interview, 159-164; Bull's-Eye Worksheet, 170-171; case example of, 158-172; CPAT used in, 164; dealing with self-blame in, 169, 170; follow-up care for, 165-172; identifying traumas for, 156-157; observer self and, 166-169; overview of, 155-158; planning and providing treatments, 164; present-moment experience in, 165-166; Response Able exercise, 170; self-stories used in, 168-169; summary of, 172-173; values connection, 170-171; victimized patients and, 155-156
treatments: for alcohol/drug abuse, 112-116; for anxiety and depression, 145-149; for chronic disease patients, 94-100; for

chronic pain patients, 124-134; tools for planning and providing, 7, 62, 74-82, 83; for trauma patients, 164
trigger questions, 66, 67
Twain, Mark, 155

U

unwillingness, 121, 135. *See also* willingness
unworkable change agenda, 41-42
unworkable rules: chronic disease interventions and, 94-95; chronic pain interventions and, 127-129; provider wellness interventions and, 199-201; stepping back from, 54-56, 79, 94-95, 127-129, 199-201; stuckness in, 34

V

values: action consistent with, 50-52, 78-79; alcohol/drug abuse patients and, 115-116; chronic disease patients and, 95-97, 98-100; disconnection from, 32; discrepancy between behavior and, 49-50, 97; identification of, 49, 95-96; professional and personal assessment of, 197-199; provider wellness and, 195-199, 203; strengthening connection with, 48-50, 78; trauma interventions and, 170-171
Velcro exercise, 56, 199-200

violence: victims of, 155-156. *See also* trauma interventions
vitality, 44-45
Vowles, Kevin, 4

W

Web resources, 7, 40, 62
wellness interventions. *See* provider wellness interventions

willingness, 56-57; modeling for chronic pain patients, 121. *See also* acceptance
Witness technique. *See* Be a Witness technique
work questions, 71, 72
workability, 42; assessment of, 42-44; interview questions about, 66, 67; vitality and, 44-45. *See also* Three-T and Workability Questions